# Hearing Disorders Handbook

Maurice H. Miller, Ph.D.
Jerome D. Schein, Ph.D.

*Professors Emeritus,*
*New York University*

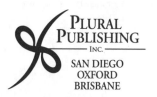

PLURAL
PUBLISHING
INC.
SAN DIEGO
OXFORD
BRISBANE

5521 Ruffin Road
San Diego, CA 92123

e-mail: info@pluralpublishing.com
Web site: http://www.pluralpublishing.com

49 Bath Street
Abingdon, Oxfordshire OX14 1EA
United Kingdom

**Library of Congress Cataloging-in-Publication Data:**

Miller, Maurice H., 1930-
  Hearing disorders handbook / Maurice H. Miller and Jerome D. Schein.
      p. ; cm.
  Includes bibliographical references and index.
  ISBN-13: 978-1-59756-282-9 (alk. paper)
  ISBN-10: 1-59756-282-3 (alk. paper)
  1.  Hearing disorders—Handbooks, manuals, etc.
  [DNLM: 1.  Hearing Disorders. 2.  Rehabilitation of Hearing
Impaired—methods. 3.  Vestibular Diseases.  WV 270 M649h 2008]
  I. Schein, Jerome Daniel. II. Title.
    RF290.M55 2008
    617.8—dc22

                                                        2008000320

# Hearing Disorders Handbook

Brad A. Stach
Editor-in-Chief for Audiology

# CONTENTS

*Preface*                                                              *vii*

*Acknowledgments*                                                       *xii*

**SECTION 1:** Introduction to Hearing                                    **1**
                and Vestibular Disorders
                1.1 Endogenous Etiology                                    17
                1.2 Exogenous Etiology                                     67
                1.3 Multiple Etiology                                      91
                1.4 Vestibular Disorders                                  147
**SECTION 2:** Management Options                                        **161**
                2.1 Amplification                                        165
                2.2 Cochlear Implants                                    181
                2.3 Strategies to Compensate                             201
                    for Hearing Loss
**SECTION 3:** Demographic, Social and                                   **221**
                Economic Aspects

*Author Index*                                                          *239*
*Subject Index*                                                         *255*

# PREFACE

*Hearing Disorders Handbook* (HDH) provides descriptions of hearing and vestibular disorders, their frequency of occurrence, etiology, diagnosis, and management. It seeks the perspectives of the diverse disciplines that make up the typical hearing rehabilitation team—disciplines that include audiology, otology, speech-language pathology, and the related fields of education, genetics, pediatrics, and psychology.

HDH does not replace traditional textbooks, lectures, or practicums. While striving to be comprehensive, HDH organizes its contents—whether of a particular disorder, symptom, or diagnostic and management procedure—comprehensively and concisely. This approach fulfills the original intent of handbooks: *to contain information in a volume small enough to be held in the hand*.

The concepts of comprehensiveness and conciseness grow more timely as the flood of information contiues to increase.[1] Because so much is written and continues to emerge, both experts and novices need the means of quickly and accurately winnowing the wheat from the chaff. In so doing, HDH guides readers through the bewildering amount of material about hearing and vestibular disorders.

## ORGANIZATION OF HDH

HDH divides into three main sections:

## Section 1. Introduction to Hearing and Vestibular Disorders

The first three subsections divide entries for hearing disorders by their causes: 1.1. Endogenous Etiology, 1.2. Exogenous Etiology, and 1.3. Multiple Etiology. Discussion of each disorder takes up its frequency of occurrence, etiology, diagnosis, and management.

The fourth subsection (1.4) concerns vestibular disorders, which organizes its entries by symptoms. The discussions of the cardinal symptoms replicate the order for hearing disorders; that is, frequency of occurrence, etiology, diagnosis, and management.

Any question about including a section on vestibular disorders in HDH should be allayed by considerations of the nature of the disorders and their interrelatedness. Factors affecting one system often impinge on the functioning of the other; for example, in patients with suspected cases of acoustic neuroma and those with Meniere's syndrome. Because many hearing disorders are also accompanied by vestibular symptoms, clinicians need information about both.[2]

## Section 2. Management Options

The sections augment specific discussions of management within each disorder and symptom. They present management options that apply generally to treatment of hearing and vestibular disorders. Its subsections are: 2.1, Amplification, 2.2, Cochlear Implants, and 2.3, Strategies to Compensate for Hearing Loss.

## Section 3. Demographic, Social, and Economic Aspects

This section addresses the principal consequences of hearing and vestibular disorders. It aims to place these disorders in their rightful position among diseases that most pervasively and significantly affect health and quality of life. It assesses the social-economic toll that hearing and vestibular disorders levy on affected individuals and their families, highlighting information and relationships that can be useful in researching and planning.

## INFORMATION RESOURCES

For readers seeking more information about a particular topic or disorder, HDH provides references to original print and electronic sources. These supplement the material condensed to fulfill the objective pf concision.

Recently, journals have appeared exclusively on the Internet. One such is Public Library of Science (PLoS Med), a nonprofit organization that supports an open-access, peer-reviewed source of articles related to medicine.[3] PLoS Med appears monthly. Being new, its value remains to be assessed by the professionals who access it.

For descriptions of extremely rare conditions that are not covered in HDH and for the most recent information about those that are represented, readers should consult the Internet. The National Center on Low Incidence Disabilities[4] and Online Mendelian Inheritance in Man[5] are particularly useful sources of current information. In addition, the National Institute of Deafness and Other Communicative Disorders[6] periodically posts notices about disorders associated with hearing loss.

Organizations specific to particular disorders are mentioned within each entry. Among organizations that address hearing and vestibular disorders broadly are the following: Association of Late Deafened Adults,[7] Hearing Loss Association of America,[8] League for the Hard of Hearing,[9] and National Association of the Deaf.

## EDITING NOTES

In multiauthored articles, only the first three authors are noted. If there are more than three authors, the abbreviation et al. ("and others") follows the third author's name. As the purpose of the citation is to enable readers to locate a reference, this limitation should not prove a hindrance to bibliographic searches.

Terminology respects the sources cited. So, for example, the terms deaf appears in the discussion when that is the designation chosen by the referenced source. Otherwise, HDH writes hearing loss or the even broader hearing impairment as appropriate to a discussion's context.

## CAUTIONARY NOTICE

The information contained in HDH does not stand in lieu of competent professional counsel. No individual should rely on HDH to determine any medical or related professional treatment. HDH makes no claims for infallibility, though it strives to ensure that all of its contents reflect accurately the state of knowledge about hearing disorders.

Aside from organizing references for easy access, HDH is mindful that the plethora of research publications contain many that are based on weak methodology and, indeed, may present fraudulent conclusions.[10] With respect to such pitfalls, HDH cannot guarantee that all materials to which it directs readers are valid. Such an objective would be beyond its scope. HDH does, however, avoid citing obviously suspect publications. To that end, HDH should provide useful access to the vast literature on hearing and vestibular disorders and stimulate its appreciation.

## REFERENCES

1. Dyson F. Our biotech future. *New York Review of Books.* 2007;54(12):4–7.
2. American Speech-Language-Hearing Association. Role of audiologists in vestibular and balance rehabilitation: Position statement, guidelines, and technical report. *Asha.* 1999;41(suppl 19): 13–22.
3. Public Library of Medicine. Retrieved October 2004 from http://journals.plos.org/plosmedicine

4. National Center on Low-Incidence Disabilities. Retrieved from http://www.nclid.unco.edu
5. Online Mendelian Inheritance in Man. Retrieved 2007 from http://www.ncbi.nlm.nih.gov/omim
6. National Institute on Deafness and Other Communicative Disorders. Retrieved May 2007 from http://www.nidcd.gov
7. Association of Late Deafened Adults. Access http://www.shhh.org
8. Hearing Loss Association of America. Access http://www.alda.org
9. League for the Hard of Hearing. Access at http://www.lhh.org
10. Ioannidis JPA. *Why most published research findings are false.* Retrieved August 2005 from http://journals.plos.org/plosmedicine

# ACKNOWLEDGMENTS

We wish to express our appreciation to the following persons, without whose generous assistance this work would have been difficult, if not impossible:

A. K. Lalwani, M.D., Mendik Foundation Professor and Chairman of the Department of Otolaryngology, New York University School of Medicine;

Joseph Montano, Ed.D., Director of Communication Disorders at New York Hospital Cornell Weil School of Medicine;

Caroline Young, JD, MLIS and other members of the Library Staff of the NYU Medical Center Library; and

our wives, Anita R. Miller and Enid G. Wolf-Schein.

Maurice H. Miller
Jerome D. Schein
March 2008

# SECTION 1

# Introduction to Hearing and Vestibular Disorders

The first three subsections of Section 1 classify hearing disorders broadly by their etiology, whereas the final subsection focuses on vestibular symptoms.

The classification of hearing disorders distributes them as endogenous (genetic), exogenous (acquired), and mixed or undetermined etiology. A fourth category considers vestibular symptoms. The onset of these conditions may occur congenitally or in subsequent years. If onset is postnatal, the cause may still be genetic, and genetic causes may be either inherited or acquired as mutations in utero.[1]

## 1.1 ENDOGENOUS ETIOLOGY

Genetic causes of hearing loss broadly divide into syndromic and nonsyndromic.[2] A syndrome is a set of symptoms that occur together; for example, Alport syndrome consists of congenital hearing loss and renal dysfunction. Nonsyndromic conditions only have a single consistent symptom; for example, Scheibe aplasia in Section 1.3.

Syndromic etiologies account for about one-third of endogenous conditions, and the nonsyndromic hearing conditions

1

and those of mixed or undetermined etiology, taken together, account for approximately two-thirds of the remainder of genetic causes.[3]

These approximations will change depending on the populations studied, the geographic areas sampled, the time period when they are assessed, and the samples' composition by age, gender, race, and other pertinent factors.

## 1.2  EXOGENOUS ETIOLOGY

Disorders resulting from nongenetic or environmental causes appear in this chapter. Congenital hearing losses can present diagnostic difficulties because they might be genetic, arise from damage in utero, or due to harm at birth or shortly after, as in cases of prematurity.[4]

## 1.3  MULTIPLE ETIOLOGY

Some disorders have more than one likely cause or result from a confluence of factors—a combination of genetic and environmental factors. They may have both dominant and recessive transmissions or may result from chromosomal anomalies, most of which are nonheritable. The etiology of other disorders simply remains in doubt.[5]

Tinnitus—a phenotype with potentially numerous causes —exemplifies an instance of mixed etiology. In presbycusis, identifying a single cause would not reflect the possibility, if not certainty, that numerous events and causal agents account for observed hearing impairments. CHARGE association and the autoimmune disorders illustrate others whose etiology has not achieved scientific consensus. Some conditions might eventually prove to be variations or incomplete expressions of a single etiology, which may account for some of the aplasias and dysplasias now considered separate syndromes. For those reasons, then, the inclusion of a condition in Section 3.1 should be considered subject to change as more research establishes their etiology.

## Criteria for Including Disorders in HDH

To eliminate entries of disorders with little or no relevance to hearing and vestibular rehabilitation, only those in which the hearing loss and/or vestibular disorders are consistent components are included in Sections 1. 1 and 1.2. The determination of "consistent component" remains unquantified; it rests on sometimes sparse epidemiologic research, with vague accounts of the frequency of occurrence of the syndrome itself, let alone its separate components.

As examples, Duane and Behcet syndromes are not included in HDH because hearing loss does not appear to be integral to them, though instances have been reported of their conjoint occurrence. These two disorders largely consist of ophthalmic anomalies, in the former,[6] and vascular inflammation, in the latter.[7] Among instances that are included in Sections 3.1 and 3.2 are those that predispose to hearing loss, as in many of the aplasias and dysplasias, as well as those in which hearing loss is a consistent component.

# ORGANIZATION WITHIN SECTION 1

Throughout Section 1, the discussions that follow each brief description of a condition fall under one of four rubrics: Frequency of Occurrence, Etiology, Diagnosis, and Management. These groupings facilitate comparisons between the conditions as well as uniformly ordering the information about each.

## Frequency of Occurrence

Numerous nongenetic causes of hearing disorders occur over an individual's life span. Congenital hearing loss occurs in about 1 to 2 per 1,000 live births.[8] Exogenous factors probably account for approximately half of them.[9] About one out of 1,000 children in the United States is born with a hearing loss so severe that, if not detected before the child's second birthday, could interfere in their development of speech and language.[10]

Myriad causes can account for hearing loss.[11] Of genetic hearing losses, about a third are syndromic; nonsyndromic hearing losses occur in about 1 per 2,000 live births.[12]

Endogenous and exogenous hearing losses are roughly divided equally in occurrence.[13] However, the incidence of endogenous causes in congenital onsets has been placed as high as 60% or higher.[14] Some degree of hearing loss—from mild to profound—is theoretically due to genetic factors in an estimated 1 in 500 live births.[15]

The incidence of late-onset hearing loss increases markedly with age. Although some of these losses appear to have an entirely or partially genetic basis, the majority of hearing losses occurring postnatally are due to environmental factors.

Rates of incidence and prevalence of many of the conditions listed in HDH are often based on series of cases in a single hospital or clinic. Although these estimates may be expressed as rates per thousand or higher, they are often derived from samples of fewer than a hundred cases. For example, one large sampling of children with hearing loss found that those due to Pendred and Usher syndromes occurred more frequently in England than in South Australia, whereas those due to Waardenburg syndrome were more prevalent in South Australia than in England.[16] Similar findings for hearing loss in various geographic areas have been reported.

To avoid misleading readers by emphasizing their often tenuous bases, HDH precedes most quoted rates by modifiers like "about," "estimated," "approximately," and so forth. By so doing, this editorial practice makes it clear that these numbers often result from educated guesses, not actual counts, and that all are subject to changing conditions within the populations for which the estimates are provided.

## Etiology

Molecular biology, the science and technology that unpacks the genetic code, has honed our knowledge of genetic factors and enhanced the determination of the extent to which a hearing loss is inherited or acquired. It provides incisive diagnostic techniques.[17]

Although molecular biology has made giant strides in solving questions of genetic transmission, its analyses of the etiology of conditions with significant hearing loss remain incomplete. This means that attribution of a condition to a genetic or non-genetic origin will sometimes be speculative. Nonetheless, it has been urged that a genetic basis be investigated in all hearing disorders whose etiologies are not established.[18]

## Diagnosis

Ample texts provide information about diagnostic audiologic procedures.[19-21] When special procedures are indicated by a condition—as in diagnosis of early childhood hearing loss—some details are provided. These direct readers' attention to special points and specific resources pertinent to a particular condition; for example, auditory neuropathy.[22]

In most instances of recessive inheritance, the family history will be negative for the disorder. A diagnostician must often probe several prior generations to find an additional relevant case. The search for such a connection in many cases may prove to be worth pursuing.[23]

Although clinicians have acquired numerous diagnostic tools in recent years, they do not substitute for a clinician's skill and assiduous probing.[24] In addition to other examinations, genetic counseling has been recommended in all cases of hearing impairment because determining a genetic basis for patients' hearing losses can provide valuable clues for treatment and, in some cases, may avoid an unnecessary death, as in Jervell and Lange-Nielsen syndrome.

## Infant Screening

Neonatal and infant screening have been widely adopted in the United States to identify hearing losses. The 2000 statement by the Joint Committee on Infant Hearing (JCIH) recommended audiologic screening for infants with one or more specified risk factors (e.g., a birthweight less than 1500 grams, infection by bacterial meningitis, and malformations of the external ear).[25] These criteria for examination, however, resulted in large numbers of infants with hearing impairments going undetected. The emphasis has shifted from high-risk inventories to Universal Newborn Hearing Screening.[26] JCIH now recommends procedures that should be performed within 48 hours of birth and before discharge from a hospital, and it urges that when amplification is appropriate it should be fitted within one month of diagnosis.[27]

Otoacoustic emissions (OAE) provide an objective, easily performed means of detecting hearing loss in newborns. It reflects cochlear outer-hair cell functioning. Because it fails to identify such conditions as auditory neuropathy for which auditory brainstem response (ABR) and immittance testing are necessary, it should be only one component of an early identification program.[28,29]

Since 1995, seven New York regional hospitals have been studying two procedures for newborn hearing screening.[30] The first method (OAE) projects low-to-moderate clicks into the neonate's ear. The second method (ABR) attaches electrodes to the neonate's scalp to measure brain activity in response to auditory stimuli sounded.[31]

For children 2.5 to 5 years of age and older, conditioning techniques have an established role in auditory assessment. Behavioral assessment procedures have been found to be ineffective in children less than 2 years of age.[32,33] Conditioned play audiometry (CPA) reinforces the child's correct responses with words of praise and smiles and is considered the most consistent behavioral technique to determine ear-specific and frequency-specific hearing thresholds of children 2.5 years of age and older. However, its use is dependent on the abilities of the person conducting the test. Examiner bias in judging responses also can be a problem. Less examiner-dependent tests include the following:[34]

■ Visual Reinforcement Audiometry (VRA), originally termed Conditioned Orientation Audiometry, attempts to condition auditory responses to visual stimuli using lighted toys. It yields reliable results with 90% of normally hearing and hearing-impaired children between 12 and 30 months of age.

■ Tangible Reinforcement Operant Conditioning Audiometry (TROCA) automatically dispenses an item such as candy or a trinket when the child responds to a sound initially presented in a sound field and later presented through earphones. Valid results have been reported with developmentally delayed children 2 to 4 years of age.

Children who fail initial screening tests should have complete audiologic examinations in the subsequent 3 months, in order to detect false positives. The next step is determining a cause. Testing the parents' DNA may find genes associated with hearing loss, establishing a causative link. A thorough prenatal history can point to potential factors that may have contributed to the childhood hearing loss.

Differentiating endogenous from exogenous causal factors offers a significant challenge to diagnosticians. Pitfalls remain, therefore, on the path to a definitive diagnosis of the etiology of a hearing loss. Even the subtle manifestation of mild hearing losses and those limited to one part of the frequency range warrant audiologic testing of all relatives of a patient with the loss. Parents often express an interest in knowing the likelihood that other offspring will have hearing loss, clearly indicating the need for referral to a genetic counselor.[35]

The American College of Medical Genetics offers evaluation guidelines to determine the etiology of individual cases.[36] The cause of a hearing loss can be complex, making definitive diagnoses difficult. It may not become apparent until later childhood or adulthood, even though it is genetic. Because mutations in several different genes are associated with hearing loss, it is possible that a person will not necessarily inherit a hearing loss even though both of the person's parents have had hearing losses.[37] This happens when the parents' hearing losses result from different genetic causes.

An inherited syndrome may only be partially expressed (referred to as incomplete penetrance). In addition, an individual's hearing loss may have both genetic and environmental causes: the latter triggering the former (see, for example, Alport syndrome). Such complications prompt a caution against too easy adoption of a causal basis for a congenital hearing loss.[14]

Another caveat: Investigating the potential genetic basis for a hearing loss may arouse sensitivities in those being investigated. Parents of deaf children often make genetic counselors aware of the delicate nature of inquiries into their heritage by their reluctance to participate in extensive questioning about themselves and their relatives.[38] Empathy for their feelings, on the other hand, should not curtail efforts to determine whether or not a genetic basis for a hearing loss accounts for it. What is more, uncovering a genetic cause can be critical, as noted in syndromes like Alport and Jervell and Lange-Nielsen— syndromes in which disorders that comprise them might go unnoticed and, therefore, unmanaged and result in serious complications and possibly death.

## Management

The selection and fitting of hearing aids is the primary rehabilitative tool for the overwhelming majority of persons with varying degrees of hearing loss. Section 3.1 discusses amplification in depth, and Section 3.2 provides information about cochlear implants.

Public Health Service guidelines propose six essential principles of effective early intervention in treatment of infants and young children with hearing losses:

1. Developmental timing
2. Program intensity

3. Direct learning
4. Program breadth and flexibility
5. Recognition of individual differences
6. Environmental support and family involvement.[39]

During their early years, frequent audiologic evaluations are advised for all children with hearing loss. Periodic examinations—at least annually—should be conducted for children with established hearing losses and for those whose hearing loss occurs later. Studies of hearing loss due to maternal rubella, for example, often show further reductions in hearing ability from childhood to adulthood.

Monitoring the affected child enables the clinician to note the course of hearing loss, which in some cases may fluctuate and in others may continue to decline. Attending to the other aspects of the syndrome can detect problems emerging from another component of the syndrome—problems that might be life-threatening. Alport syndrome, for example, includes renal disease the presence of which can result in fatal consequences. As another example, persons with Usher syndrome usually suffer exacerbations of visual loss over many years, so treatment must be adjusted to accommodate to these changes.

Treatment and monitoring receive attention specific for each disorder as that disorder is discussed. These specifics focus on aspects beyond those covered in Section 2, Management Options, which summarizes general procedures and instrumentation that apply across conditions.

Amplification and cochlear implants are the treatments of choice for most disorders that involve hearing loss, but many hearing disorders have requirements that differ from the others in selection of instruments. For example, the differences in prescribing hearing aids for infants and elderly persons are discussed in their respective places as well as in Sections 2.1 and 2.2. Similarly, amplification for patients with unilateral hearing losses raise particular issues distinct from those applicable to patients with bilateral hearing losses.

The advent of cochlear implants has added substantially to the treatment options available to hearing rehabilitation. Section 2.2 contains an extensive discussion of the preconditions that must be met before choosing this treatment, the choices of instruments, postoperative treatment, and results of this procedure.

Instrumentation alone does not illustrate the extent of strategies and tactics for the rehabilitation of hearing losses. Section 2.3, therefore, presents a host of noninstrumental approaches.

Most sensorineural hearing losses are considered irreversible regardless of their etiology. However, there are exceptions.[40]

Efforts are underway to alter genetic conditions that lead to hearing loss.[41] Traditionally, clinicians only deal with the consequences of a genetic condition, not offering cures but providing, as appropriate, amplification, cochlear implants, and compensation strategies. Recently, researchers have examined the possibilities of stem cells to reverse the inherent cellular defect(s) that lead to hearing loss. They have isolated cochlear stem cells in animals that are primed to develop into ear-related tissue, and hypothesize that the cochlea also harbors neural precursor cells that may be able to regenerate hair cells. They see the ability of cultured mouse stem cells to form cell spheres as contributing supporting evidence for this hypothesis, a first step in designing gene therapy.[42] Further challenges to the belief that CNS tissue cannot be regenerated have arisen from research limiting the effects of traumatic brain injury.[43]

## Gene Manipulation as Therapy

Study of gene therapy for Usher syndrome, among others, has potential for altering the course of this disorder, if not eliminating it. Gene manipulation will be used increasingly to prevent various syndromic and nonsyndromic causes of hearing loss. The work of the National Institutes of Health on connexin 26 gene, a major cause of hereditary hearing loss, is an example.

Although it is a long stretch from animal studies to human applications, this research bears watching.[44]

For the present, treatment for most genetic forms of hearing loss does not differ substantially from that for exogenous etiologies. Relieving the developmental and communicative delays caused by reduced or absent hearing ability devolve on education, counseling, and amplification, as outlined in Section 3. The earlier such treatment is undertaken, the better the outcome is likely to be.

Hearing rehabilitation should be considered as an ongoing process that is available throughout the patient's life. Monitoring following the initiation of treatment should be sought in every case of hearing loss because changes often occur in the nature and severity of the condition for which treatment was originally designed and other disorders may emerge.

Follow-up recommendations, as with those for initial treatment, tend to be similar across disorders. One recommendation that recurs is to attend to the vision of anyone suffering a loss of hearing. From codependence for distant communication and alerting, the hearing loss shifts more toward visual dependence. This means an increased use of the visual system, to the extent that it remains intact. For that reason, testing the adequacy of vision and making corrections as appropriate are critical to hearing rehabilitation.

## SECTION 1.4  VESTIBULAR DISORDERS

The approach to vestibular disorders in this Section shifts from organization by underlying causes to categorization by symptoms. Within each symptom subcategory, the presentations follow the order for hearing disorders: description, frequency of occurrence, etiology, diagnosis, and management, insofar as pertinent information on each allows.

The decision to organize this Section around symptoms recognizes that the etiologies of vestibular disorders are either so diverse or indeterminate as to make such a classification scheme of little value. The major vestibular disorders of vertigo,

dizziness, disequilibrium, and nystagmus receive specific attention. Within the balance disorders, emphasis is placed on the
distinction between dizziness and vertigo—a critical distinction
both for management of vestibular disorders and also for hearing syndromes that include them, like Meniere's disease.

## TERMINOLOGY

Professional publications need to be clear about their terms of
reference, but the typical English dictionary is not an adequate
resource to depend on for definitions pertinent to hearing and
vestibular disorders. In HDH the need for care in defining
terms is great because so many different professions relate to
hearing rehabilitation.

### Hearing Terms

The most general term for all types and degrees of hearing disorder is *hearing impairment. Hearing loss* refers to any decrement in the degree of hearing ability.

   Degrees of hearing loss may be rendered as mild, moderate, severe, or profound. The term *hard of hearing* covers
degrees of hearing from less than normal through severe—
approximately 25 to 90 dB. HDH reserves *deaf* for the extreme
degree of hearing loss, usually severe to profound, with the
audiometric level for the average at 500, 1000, and 2000 Hz
equal to or above 90 dB.[45]

   Specific definitions of these terms differ among those
using them. HDH only uses *deaf* and *hard of hearing* when
citing studies that specify these terms. Otherwise, HDH uses
either *hearing loss* or *hearing impairment*, as applicable, to
avoid confusion.

### Genetic Terms

Two other terms common to genetics are sequence and syndrome. A sequence is a series of disorders occurring from a sin-

gle developmental defect; for example, Pierre-Robin sequence (see Section 1.3). It differs from syndrome in that syndrome refers to a group of related symptoms arising from a single genetic condition; for example, Alport syndrome (see Section 1.1).

# REFERENCES

1. Nance WE. The epidemiology of hereditary deafness: the impact of connexion 26 on the size and structure of the deaf community. In: Van Cleve JV, ed. *Genetics, Disability, and Deafness.* Washington, DC: Gallaudet University Press; 2004.

2. Gorlin RJ, Toricello HV, Cohen MM. *Hereditary Hearing Loss and Its Syndromes.* New York, NY: Oxford University Press; 1995.

3. *Proceedings of the National Academy of Science.* Retrieved May 2007 from http://www.pnas.org/cgi/content/abstract/104/2/1337

4. Steel KP. A new era in the genetics of deafness. *N Engl J Med.* 1998;339(21):1545–1547.

5. Denoyelle F, Linada-Grenada G, Plauchie H, et al. Connexin 26 gene linked to a dominant deafness. *Nature.* 1998;393:319–320.

6. Ro A, Chernoff G, MacRae D, et al. Auditory function in Duane's retraction syndrome. *Am J Ophthalmol.* 1990;109(1):75–78.

7. Behcet's syndrome. Retrieved April 2007 from http://www.nlm.nih.gov/medlineplus/behcetssyndrome.html

8. Statement of the American College of Medical Genetics, January 2000.

9. Dionisopoulos T, Williams HB. *Congenital Anomalies of the Ear, Nose and Throat.* New York, NY: Oxford University Press; 1997.

10. Rapin I. Conductive hearing loss effects on children's language and scholastic skills. A review of the literature. *Ann Otol Rhinol Laryngol.* 1979;88:3–12.

11. Post JC. Genetic principles. In: Wetmore RF, Muntz JR, Merrill TJ, eds. *Principles and Practice Pathways.* New York, NY: Thieme; 2000.

12. Online Mendelian Inheritance in Man. Retrieved January 2007 from http://www.ncbi.nlm.nih.gov/omim

13. Brookhouser PE, Smith SD. Genetic hearing loss. In Bailey EJ, ed. *Otolaryngology and Head and Neck Surgery.* 2nd ed. Philadelphia, Pa: Lippincott; 1998.

14. Dagan O, Avraham KB. The complexity of hearing loss from a genetics perspective. In: Van Cleve JV, ed. *Genetics, Disability, and Deafness.* Washington, DC: Gallaudet University Press; 2004.

15. Morton NE. Genetic epidemiology of hearing impairment. *Ann New York Acad Sci.* 1991;630:16–31.

16. Fraser GR. *The Causes of Profound Deafness in Childhood.* Baltimore, Md: Johns Hopkins University Press; 1976.

17. Grundfast KM, Atwood JL, Chuong D. Genetics and molecular biology of deafness. *Otolaryngol Clin North Am.* 1999;32(6): 1067–1088.

18. Keats BJB. Genetic intervention and hearing loss. In: Roeser RJ, Valente H, Hosford-Dunn H. *Audiology Diagnosis.* New York, NY: Thieme, 2000.

19. Katz J, ed. *Handbook of Clinical Audiology.* 5th ed. Baltimore, Md: Lippincott Williams & Wilkins; 2002.

20. Roeser RJ, Valente M, Hosford-Dunn H. *Audiology Diagnosis.* New York NY: Thieme; 2000.

21. Gelfand SA, ed. *Essentials of Audiology.* 2nd ed. New York, NY: Thieme; 2001.

22. Berlin CI, Bordelin J, St John P, et al. Reversing click polarity may uncover auditory neuropathy in infants. *Ear Hear.* 1998; 19:37–47.

23. Bussoli TJ, Steel KP. The molecular genetics of inherited deafness—current and future applications. *J Laryngol Otol.* 1998; 112(6):523–530.

24. American Speech-Language-Hearing Association. 2001. Knowledge and skills required for the practice of audiological/aural rehabilitation. Retrieved October 2001 from http://www.asha.org/policy

25. Norton SJ, Gorga MP, Widen JE, et al. Identification of neonatal hearing Impairment: evaluation of transient evoked otoacoustic emission, distortion product otoacoustic emission and auditory brainstem response test performance. *Ear Hear.* 2000;21:508–528.

26. Johnson JL, White KR, Widen JE, et al. A multicenter evaluation of how many infants with permanent hearing loss pass a

two-stage otoacoustic emissions/automated auditory brainstem response newborn hearing screening protocol. *Pediatrics*. 2005;6(3):663–672.

27. Joint Committee on Infant Hearing. JCIH position statement: principles and guidelines for early hearing detection and intervention programs. Retrieved October 27, 2007 from http://www.asha.org/docs/html/PS2007-00281.html

28. Glassman SA, Matkin ND, Sabo MP. Early identification of congenital sensorineural hearing loss. *Hear J*. 1987;40(9):13–17.

29. Harrison M, Roush J. Age of suspicion, identification and intervention for infants and young children with hearing loss: a national study. *Ear Hear*. 1996;17:55–62.

30. Spivak LG, ed. *Universal Newborn Hearing Screening*. New York, NY: Thieme; 1998.

31. Spivak LG, Prieve B, Dalzell L, et al. The New York State universal newborn hearing screening demonstration project: inpatient outcome measures. *Ear Hear*. 2000;21(2):92–103.

32. Shoup AG, Roeser RJ. Audiologic evaluation of special populations. In Roeser RJ, Valente M, Hosford-Dunn H. *Audiology Diagnosis*. New York, NY: Thieme; 2000:370–382.

33. Thompson G, Weber BA. Responses of infants and young children to behavioral observation audiometry. *J Speech Hear Dis*. 1974;39:140–147.

34. American Speech-Language-Hearing Association. Guidelines for the audiologic assessment of children from birth to 5 years of age. Retrieved November 2004 from http://www.asha.org/members/deskrefjournals/deskref/default

35. K Kitamura, KP Steel, eds. *Genetics in Otorhinolaryngology. Advances in Otorhinolaryngology*. 2000;56:275–278.

36. American College of Medical Genetics Expert Panel. Universal newborn hearing screening. *Genet Med*. 2002;2:149–150.

37. Griffith A, Yang Y, Pryor SP, et al. Cochleosaccular dysplasia associated with connexin 26 mutation in keratitis-ichthyosis-deafness syndrome. *Laryngoscope*. 2006;116(8):1404–1408.

38. Middleton A. Deaf and hearing adults' attitudes toward genetic testing for deafness. In: Van Cleve JV, ed. *Genetics, Disability, and Deafness*. Washington, DC: Gallaudet University Press; 2004.

39. Stool SE, Berg AO, Berman S, et al. Otitis media with effusion in young children. *Clinical Practice Guideline, Number 12*.

AHCPR Publication No. 94-0622. Rockville, Md: Agency for Health Care Policy and Research, Public Health Service, US Department of Health and Human Services; 1994.

40. Miller MH, Kalmon M, Fowler EP. Marked improvement in bone conduction. *Ann Otol Rhinol Laryngol.* 1957;66:981-994.

41. Lalwani AK, Mhatre AN. Cochlear gene therapy. In: Kitamura K, Steel KP, eds. *Genetics in Otorhinolaryngoly. Advances in Otorhinolaryngo*logy. Vol 56. Basel: Karger; 2000:275-278.

42. Yerulkhimovich MV, Bai L, Chen DH-C, et al. Identification and characterization of mouse cochlear stem cells. *Der Neurosciences.* 2007;29:251-260.

43. Epstein S. Early ear cell regeneration and pros and cons of implantable hearing aids. *Volta Voices.* 2007;14(95):42-43.

44. Crumling MA, Raphael Y. Manipulating gene expression in the inner ear. *Brain Res.* 2006;1091:265-269.

45. Davis H. Abnormal hearing and deafness: definitions and distinctions. In: Davis H, Silverman SR, eds. *Hearing and Deafness.* 4th ed. London, UK: Holt, Rinehart & Winston; 1978; 87-146.

# Section 1.1

# *Endogenous Etiology*

## ALPORT SYNDROME (ALP)

ALP syndrome consists of hearing loss and kidney disease. Its expression may include cataracts and bulging of the lens (lenticonus). The hearing loss is often progressive, may be both sensorineural and conductive, and usually occurs in pre-adolescence.[1]

## Frequency of Occurrence

In the United States, the prevalence of ALP is estimated to be about 1 in 5,000.[2]

## Etiology

ALP is one of several disorders that involve hearing loss and kidney dysfunction; for example, Hypoparathyroidism-Deaf-ness-Renal Dysplasia syndrome discussed below. ALP usually affects only males, as the genetic deviation is typically found on the X chromosome. However, there is a closely related form that can also affect females, in whom the symptoms are less severe and develop slower than in men.[3]

    The genetic defect causes chronic glomerulonephritis. Progressive destruction of the glomeruli leads to loss of kidney function that leads to end-stage renal disease, which may occur at any time between the teens and the fifth decade of life.

ALP has a number of expressions, one of which may be activated by a particular class of drugs (aminoglycosides) that act as medication triggers. In another variation, occurring largely in the western United States, affected persons have an onset of kidney failure in the fourth or fifth decade, followed by significant loss of hearing.[4] A further variation is Epstein syndrome, which is composed of nephritis, deafness, and macrothrombocytopathia.[5]

Although sensorineural deafness occurs frequently, but not always, in patients with ALP, it is usually not present at birth but typically is manifested in childhood or early adolescence.

## Diagnosis

ALP's earliest indication is hematuria (blood in the urine).[6] Its prompt diagnosis can avoid later complications that may be life-threatening.[7]

## Management

Treating the nephritis and being alert to medication and procedures that might initiate kidney failure can avert life-threatening complications. Surgeries to extract cataracts and repair the anterior lenticonus are therapies that can be undertaken, if needed.

The sensorineural hearing loss in ALP cannot be reversed, but the conductive component, when present, may be surgically corrected. Audiometric monitoring is essential.

# CHARCOT-MARIE-TOOTH SYNDROME (CMT)

CMT is an autosomal dominant, progressive nerve disease that causes gradual decrease of muscle function, primarily in the legs. Sensorineural hearing losses occur in some, but not all, cases.[8]

CMT is also called Hereditary Motor and Sensory Neuropathy or Peroneal Muscular Atrophy. It is named for the famous

French psychiatrist, Jean-Martin Charcot, his student, Pierre Marie, and the English physician, Howard H. Tooth.

## Frequency of Occurrence

CMT has an estimated prevalence rate of about 1 in 2,500 people in the United States.[9]

## Etiology

CMT comprises a group of disorders caused by mutations in genes that affect the normal function of the peripheral nerves —probably by a mutation in the connexin 32 gene.[10]

It typically features a hearing loss that arises in adolescence. In the absence of a hearing loss, incomplete penetrance is usually thought to explain its absence.[11]

## Diagnosis

The primary signs of CMT are peripheral neuropathy. A family history and DNA analysis may be necessary to eliminate doubts about the diagnosis.[12]

Onset of symptoms generally occurs in adolescence or early adulthood but may be delayed into later adulthood. The gradual progression of symptoms and the fact that CMT has many forms with variable expression makes diagnosis somewhat difficult, especially in the patient's early years.[13]

## Management

A thorough audiologic assessment should be made in all cases of CMT. Because the hearing loss usually occurs later in an affected individual's development, monitoring hearing is an essential component of management.

Support and continuing information for patients with CMT and their families can be obtained from the Charcot-Marie-Tooth Association.[14]

# CROUZON DISEASE (CD)

CD is characterized by craniofacial malformations, so it is also known as Craniofacial Dsyostosis. A closely related condition is Alpert syndrome (APT), which also features craniofacial dysostosis, malocclusion, and abnormalities of the limbs, such as web feet and hands.[15]

Mental retardation or learning disabilities occurs in nearly all cases of CD and APT. They also predispose to infections that lead to conductive hearing losses.

## Frequency of Occurrence

CD and APT are each estimated to occur at rates of fewer than 1 per 150,000 live births.[16]

## Etiology

CD and APT comprise ocular deformations and craniosynostosis. Affected individuals may have poor mental development and convulsions. About a third of persons with CD and APT have conductive hearing loss due to fixation of the stapes footplate and deformities of the ossicular chain.[17] Inheritance of CD and APT is due to an autosomal dominant gene or genes. In the case of APT, the mutation, which probably occurs during pregnancy, has been identified as affecting a gene on chromosome 10 that affects the encoding of fibroblast growth factor (FGFR2).[18]

## Diagnosis

The facial characteristics make the presence of these syndromes apparent. However, DNA analysis may be needed to confirm those cases in which the additional symptoms resemble those in similar syndromes.

The hearing loss is uncovered by audiologic evaluations, which should be conducted regularly in every instance of APT and CD.

## Management

The bony deformities offer little possibility of alteration, although plastic surgery may be tried.[19] The conductive aspects of the otic abnormalities may be amenable to surgery, although its outcomes are by no means certain. Appropriate amplification and audiologic rehabilitation should be prescribed when a hearing loss becomes evident.

# DIDMOAD SYNDROME

DIDMOAD syndrome derives it names from the acronym based on the initials for Diabetes Insipidus, Diabetes Mellitus, Optic Atrophy, and Deafness.[20] It consists of a number of neurologic symptoms: hearing loss, optic atrophy, and either juvenile-onset diabetes insipidus or diabetes mellitus.[21]

DIDMOAD is also known as Wolfram syndrome, named for the physician who first reported it in 1938.[22]

## Frequency of Occurrence

DIDMOAD's prevalence is estimated to be between 1 and 4 per 800,000 in the general population.[23]

## Etiology

DIDMOAD is usually classified as an autosomal recessive disorder. Although consensus favors that classification, the possibility that it or a variant of it is dominant has been posed. Also, two different genetic routes of transmission, autosomal recessive and mitochondrial, have been postulated.[24]

## Diagnosis

DIDMOAD's symptoms vary considerably. As a progressive neurodegenerative disease, it progresses slowly. The ocular defects —diminished acuity and loss of color vision—usually arise in late childhood.[25]

Only insulin-dependent diabetes mellitus and bilateral progressive optic atrophy in a child are necessary to make a presumptive diagnosis of DIDMOAD. Symptoms of diabetes insipidus and poorly controlled diabetes mellitus may be confused in its early stages. Both may be present in childhood, adolescence, or early adult life. Often, but not invariably, diabetes mellitus is detected first.

Sensorineural hearing loss, which develops in about two-thirds of those with DIDMOAD, usually is not diagnosed before the average affected patient reaches middle to late adolescence. The hearing loss tends to affect the high frequencies selectively, although its effects may be broader, as a longitudinal study of three families uncovered.[26]

## Management

Once the DIDMOAD diagnosis is established, management focuses on screening for and treating its other predictable disorders. Cases in which patients with DIDMOAD remain symptom-free between adolescence and early adulthood—though unusual—make mandatory the genetic screening of their close relatives.[27]

Treatment of DIDMOAD's complications is essential. Its complications vary considerably. In some the auditory nerve and in others the digestive system nerves are spared. However, some parts of the CNS are universally affected in DIMOAD; for example, the optic nerve and the nerves that regulate sugar metabolism usually suffer. In the end, most patients succumb to its complex of diseases before 35 years.[28]

Patients and their families may be interested in the Worldwide Society of Wolfram Syndrome Families, which maintains a Web site and provides a way of contacting others with the same disease.[29]

# HUNTER AND HURLER SYNDROMES (H/HS)

H/HS are separate but similar conditions whose principal characteristics are skeletal malformations (drawfism, hunchback), mental retardation, and sensorineural deafness.[30,31] Affected persons also tend to have cardiac anomalies, ocular defects, and decreased joint mobility, though all of the latter conditions are not necessarily found in any individual expression of the syndrome.[32]

## Frequency of Occurrence

H/HS occur rarely. They have an estimated incidence of about 1 per 10,000 births, respectively. No gender, ethnic or racial differences have been postulated.[33]

## Etiology

H/HS are metabolic disorders that lead to mucopolysaccharidosis, labeled MPS I, for Hurler and MPS 2 for Hunter. Their inheritance also differs: Hurler is autosomal recessive, and Hunter is X-linked.[1] Most of their effects become manifest in the latter months of an infant's first year, but the hearing loss is congenital. Affected children usually die within their first 10 years.

## Diagnosis

Once into the first year, the syndrome becomes apparent to clinicians familiar with H/HS. Urinalysis has characteristics that confirm the diagnosis, if it is in doubt. DNA analysis may be necessary to differentiate Hunter from Hurler syndromes in some instances.[34]

## Management

Enzyme replacement and bone-marrow transplants have been proposed for the metabolic disorders, but none appears to have been reliably successful.[35]

# HYPOPARATHYROIDISM-DEAFNESS-RENAL DYSPLASIA SYNDROME (HDR)

HDR is an autosomal dominant disorder caused by mutations of GATA3. Persons with HDR exhibit sensorineural deafness, renal dysplasia, and often mental retardation.[36] In addition to the symptoms for which it is named, HDR symptoms may include muscle aches, facial twitching, carpopedal spasm, stridor, seizures, and syncope. Affected individuals may also have a history of nasal and/or delayed speech from velopharyngeal insufficiency.

## Frequency of Occurrence

HDR is rare. Its incidence in the United States has not been determined. In Japan, a recent survey estimated it to be 7.2 cases per million. It is equally prevalent in males and females. Newborns may present with hypoparathyroidism, but HDR can appear in persons of any age.[37]

## Etiology

Thirteen different mutations were identified in patients with HDR, revealing three classes of GATA3 mutations.[38]

## Diagnosis

Differential diagnosis of HDR requires care. Chromosome band 22q11-deletion (velocardiofacial syndrome or DiGeorge syndrome) has similar characteristic physical features, but hypoparathyroidism may be the only immediately distinguishing manifestation. Typically, patients with DiGeorge syndrome are diagnosable during the first few weeks of life. Patients with autoimmune and PTH-resistance syndromes tend to present as late as adolescence. A history of radioactive iodine ablation of the thyroid for Graves' disease may predate the development of acquired hypoparathyroidism by several months.

## Management

There is presently no cure for HDR. Therapy with vitamin D should be restricted to symptomatic individuals and should be sufficient enough to relieve symptoms without normalizing serum-calcium concentrations. Treatment with hydrochloroth-iazide has been shown to be beneficial, though not curative.[39]

# JERVELL AND LANGE-NIELSEN SYNDROME

Jervell and Lange-Nielsen syndrome (JNL) presents with cardiac abnormalities characterized by a recognizable electrocardio-graphic pattern and congenital severe-to-profound hearing loss. The concurrence of deafness and heart defect was only uncovered in the mid-20th century by the two scientists who initially described it.[40]

## Frequency of Occurrence

Estimates of the prevalence of JNL place it in the rare category. In the United Kingdom, for example, its prevalence has been estimated to vary between about 1.6 and 6.0 per 100,000 children between 4 and 15 years of age. Gender also influences transmission of this genetic fault.[41]

## Etiology

The genetic inheritance of JNL is not disputed, though the nature of its etiology has not been settled finally.[42] It is hetero-geneous, and appears to result from a recessive trait.[43]

The long QT-arrhythmia syncope part of the syndrome is transmitted as an autosomal dominant trait due to mutations in the LQT1 gene KvLQT1; only one abnormal copy of the KvLQT1 gene is required to produce these findings. The deafness part of the syndrome is transmitted as an autosomal recessive trait, as both copies of the KvLQT1 gene must be abnormal in order for the hearing mechanism to be affected.[44]

Mutations in a gene that also are implicated in Ward-Romano syndrome appear to account for a sizable proportion of the instances of this syndrome. In a small number of cases, other genetic mutations also have been reported to account for this syndrome.

## Diagnosis

Because sudden death is among JNL's consequences, clinicians are strongly advised to recognize signs and symptoms associated with this syndrome. Prior to identification of JNL, an incident in which a deaf child had an attack of syncope was usually ignored, as fainting was the only symptom in addition to the hearing loss. However, if fainting were due to JLN, an EKG would display a pathognomonic pattern. Such diagnosis would, then, be potentially lifesaving. For that reason, it is recommended that all children with hearing losses be given EKGs.

## Management

Once the diagnosis has been made, treatment of the heart defect and constant alertness to signs of cardiac arrhythmia become paramount. The management of the hearing loss should be simultaneously addressed, per Section 2.

## KARTAGENER SYNDROME

Kartagener syndrome (KS) is a congenital condition first recognized in 1933.[45] It affects cilia motility, which leads to primary ciliary dyskinesia (PCD). Congenital ciliary disorders are now classified as PCD to differentiate them from those that are acquired.[46]

## Frequency of Occurrence

In the United States, the frequency of KS is estimated to be about 1 in 32,000 live births. It does not appear to favor either gender.

## Etiology

KS inheritance is autosomal recessive. Its symptoms vary widely among affected individuals.[47]

Lateral displacement of some organs (situs inversus) occurs in approximately half of PCD patients. Other KS manifestations are chronic respiratory diseases, male infertility, and secondary and recurrent otitis media. Chronic childhood infections become less frequent toward the end of KS patients' second decade, and many patients lead essentially normal adult lives.

## Diagnosis

The genetic basis can be determined by DNA analysis and detailed family history.

Otoscopic examination may expose a retracted tympanic membrane with poor or absent mobility and middle-ear effusion. Audiometric testing typically yields a flat tympanogram and bilateral conductive hearing loss. Other associated otologic disorders may include tympanosclerosis, cholesteatoma, and keratosis obturans.

## Management

Management of the otic complications focuses on the frequent bouts of otitis media. KS patients often undergo repeated tympanostomy tube insertions that are complicated by chronic suppurative otitis media.[48] The hearing loss that usually develops should be treated promptly by surgery, with appropriate amplification when indicated.[49]

# MITOCHONDRIAL DISEASE

Mitochondria disease (MitD) attacks mitochondria, which are the principal sites of adenosne triphosphate (ATP), essential genetic elements that aid energy production.

## Frequency of Occurrence

Estimates of MitD ranges from about 1 to 2 per 4,000 live births.[50]

## Etiology

All mDNA is transmitted from a child's mother; therefore, if one of her children has a genetic hearing loss due to mDNA, all of her offspring will have hearing losses due to this mutation. The mDNA mutations accumulate naturally during life and are now implicated as an important cause of normal aging.

The approximately 16,000 pairs of mitochondria have their own DNA (mDNA). Related disorders include MELAS syndrome and Mohr-Tranebjaerg syndrome. MitD has also been associated with Kearns-Sayre syndrome.[51]

## Diagnosis

Diagnosis is made by observation of patients and studying their family histories, and it is ultimately confirmed by blood tests and genetic analysis. MitD's symptoms are apparent by age 5 years. Hearing loss is common. An mDNA mutation—one in which a G instead of an A occupies position 1555 in the genome—results in severe to profound sensorineural hearing loss.

## Management

Patients with MitD are unusually sensitive to aminoglycosides. In some patients, the hearing loss does not occur until triggered by exposure to aminoglycosides, like neomycin and kanamycin.[52]

Physicians who are treating patients with this mutation may avoid a hearing loss due to medication by seeking an alternative, nonototoxic antibiotic. The treating physician, however, is not likely to have such knowledge, unless a detailed genetic investigation has been made and the mitochondrial inheritance identified. However, certain mutations appear to predict the ototoxicity of the aminoglycosides, reducing the risk of hearing loss from these medications.[53]

## MOHR-TRANEBJAERG SYNDROME

Mohr-Tranebjaerg syndrome (MTS) is characterized by childhood onset of sensorineural deafness, progressive dystonia, spasticity, dysphagia, and optic atrophy.[54] It may also include psychiatric symptoms, cognitive impairment, and behavioral problems. It may also be listed as Dystonia-Deafness syndrome. See also Mitochondrial Disease and X-linked deafness.

MTS was first described in 1960 by two Swedish investigators, who believed it was nonsyndromic.[55] However, later research by Tranebjaerg found otherwise, which accounts for its current designation.[56]

## Frequency of Occurrence

The National Institutes of Health lists it as a rare disease that probably affects fewer than 200,000 people in the U. S. population, or a prevalence of fewer than about 1 per 15,000. For Europe, a consortium estimates the incidence of MTS as less than 3 per 15,000.[57]

## Etiology

MTS is an X-linked genetic mutation. A mutation in the mitochondria reputedly causes this syndrome. It is a multifocal, progressive neurodegeneration that affects portions of the CNS due to a genetic defect located in the mitochondria DDP1.[58] Absence of DDP1 impairs specific mitochondrial functions leading to degeneration of nerve cells.

The accompanying spinocerebellar degeneration resembles Fredreich ataxia and Jensen syndrome,[59,60] and it has also been suggested that the progressive hearing loss constitutes a true auditory neuropathy.[61]

## Diagnosis

Except for early-onset deafness, all other manifestations of MTS vary in their degree of severity and clinical course. As an X-linked disorder, females are not particularly affected, although carrier females have shown signs of minor neuropathy and mild hearing impairment.[62]

## Management

There is no specific treatment for MTS, as is the case with other mitochondrial disorders. Early intervention to overcome the hearing loss is key to limiting speech and language delays (see Section 2).

## MELAS SYNDROME

The initials of MELAS create the acronym for this disorder: Mitochondrial myopathy, Encephalopathy, Lactic Acidosis, and Stroke. It is a progressively degenerative nerve disorder. Typical patients present with the named features, plus seizures, diabetes mellitus, and hearing loss. Results of a Japanese study suggest that MELAS affects inner-ear structures causing deafness.[63] About 1 in 4 of MELAS patients have a sensorineural hearing loss.

## Frequency of Occurrence

The incidence of MELAS appears to involve racial factors. It may be less frequent among African-Americans than among Whites in the United States. In Finland, it has been estimated to occur at a remarkably high rate of 102 per 10,000 adults compared to a prevalence estimate for Northern England of less than 1 per 10,000.[64]

## Etiology

MELAS affects CNS, skeletal musculature, eye and heart muscles, and the cochlea. The gene mutation responsible results from disturbance of mitochondrial transfer. However, all of the pathology has not been explained. For example, strokes may be secondary to alterations in nitric-oxide homeostasis caused by microvascular damage. Research concludes that the genetic mutations are heteroplasmic, reflecting varying involvement of portions of mutated mitochondrial DNA.

Another cause of a hearing loss in MELAS may be cochlear damage that resembles presbycusis, in that it is generally symmetrical, gradual, and first affects the higher frequencies.[65] Other studies have concluded the hearing loss in MELAS is associated with mitochondrial mutations.[66,67]

## Diagnosis

The likelihood of strokes, followed by hemiplegia, hemianopia, and possible premature death make an accurate diagnosis important. A muscle biopsy for mitochondrial enzymes and DNA analysis may open a diagnosis to question, rather than resolving doubts.

MELAS is usually expressed fully from 4 to 15 years of age, although it has been reported in infants. Its onset usually appears with muscle weakness, low tolerance for exercise, and low energy reserves. It has also been associated with progressive mental retardation and other CNS difficulties.

## Management

MELAS patients require medical care. Medications, moderate exercise programs, and changes in diet may affect the course of aspects of the syndrome beneficially, although such programs lack compelling research support.[68]

Treatment for the hearing loss does not differ from that for other sensorineural losses. Referral to a genetic counselor is recommended for the patient with MELAS and family members.

# NEUROFIBROMATOSIS

Neurofibromatosis has at least two variations. Of interest to hearing rehabilitation is Type 2 (NFT-2), an autosomal dominant genetic disorder that features schwannomas and intracranial tumors among its consistent conditions. von Recklinghausen's disease is an alternative name for this neurogenetic disorder. Its popular name is Elephant Man's disease.

There are two related subtypes of Neurofibromatosis. Type 1 largely involves the peripheral nerves, and Type 2 (NFT-2) mostly attacks the CNS.[69]

## Frequency of Occurrence

Type 1 is more common than Type 2. The latter type may give rise to acoustic tumors, which in turn cause hearing loss. The possibility exists of two additional phenotypes of even rarer occurrence than Types 1 and 2.[70] NFT-2 is extremely rare, having an estimated incidence between 1 per 50,000 and 120,000 births, compared to an incidence for Type 1 of about 1 per 3,000 births.[71]

Of patients who are affected by NFT-2, hearing loss is found in about half. The incidence rate of NFT-2 does not appear to be affected by gender, race, or ethnicity.[72]

## Etiology

The NFT-2 gene has been located on chromosome 22. When normal, the gene produces a tumor-suppressing protein.[73]

In NFT-2, neurofibromas tend to form in adolescence. The nVIII tumors are the cause of the approximately half of hearing losses in patients with NFT-2. The tumors may be bilateral or unilateral, with the bilateral form of tumors occurring in about three-quarters of the cases with hearing loss.

## Diagnosis

The National Institutes of Health have provided criteria for the diagnosis of NFT-1.[74] Similar diagnostic criteria for NFT-2 have been promised. Family history and physical examination, which should include computerized tomography (CT) and magnetic-resonance imaging (MRI) of the CNS, usually resolve any diagnostic confusion.

Some signs of this condition are often apparent at birth, and almost certainly by the time an affected child attains 10 years of age. The hearing loss and tinnitus become manifest by adolescence. Diagnosis of NFT-2 is possible by amniocentesis. A rare case of NFT-2 led to deafness in a teenage boy, suggesting that this condition may not be apparent until the second or third decade.[75]

## Management

Amplification can be difficult because of the swelling due to tumors. In these cases, treatment with an implant has been developed that can be inserted into the cochlear nucleus of the brainstem to provide some useful sensory input.[76] This prosthesis is discussed further in Section 2.2.

Some medical treatments have been tried, with varying success and with an occasional danger of worsening the disease's effects.[77] The American Academy of Pediatrics Committee on Genetics recommends annual examinations, including audiometic evaluations. Periodic assessments of speech and language development are also recommended.[78]

Those interested in current updates of information and of support should contact Neurofibromatosis, Inc.[79] and Acoustic Neuroma Association.[80]

# NORRIE DISEASE (NORD)

NorD is an X-linked recessive disorder that leads to blindness in male infants at or soon after birth. It may include progressive sensorineural hearing loss, specific ocular symptoms (pseudotumor of the retina, retinal hyperplasia, hypoplasia and necrosis of the inner layer of the retina), and mental retardation.

## Frequency of Occurrence

NorD is a rare disorder that almost exclusively affects males. It occurs too infrequently to make reliable calculations of incidence rates, but these appear to be in small parts per million live births.

NorD's occurrence is not associated with any racial or ethnic group. Typically, fewer than half of patients with NorD develop progressive hearing loss, and more than half suffer developmental delays in motor-skill development.[81]

## Etiology

It is widely believed that mutations in the NDP gene cause NorD. The NDP gene provides instructions for making norrin, a protein that is involved in the establishment of a blood supply to tissues of the retina and the inner ear, and the development of some other somatic systems.

As an X-linked recessive, fathers cannot pass NorD's traits to their sons. In a tiny number of instances, carrier females have shown some retinal abnormalities and/or mild hearing loss associated with NorD, but a mutation must be present in both copies of the gene to cause the fully expressed disorder.

## Diagnosis

During the first months of life, the telltale signs of NorD can be detected by examination of the infant's retina and careful audiologic evaluation. The final diagnosis will also depend on a familial history to identify the genetic basis.

## Management

As the hearing loss in NorD occurs in the second and third decades, follow-up audiologic examinations should be undertaken on a regular basis, beginning in early childhood.

Further information about this disorder can be found by contacting the Norrie Disease Association, a voluntary not-for-profit organization dedicated to providing support and information to people with NorD and their families.[82]

## OCULO-AURICULO-VERTEBRAL SPECTRUM

OAVS is a congenital birth defect that is characterized by skull and spinal-column abnormalities. It is also known as Goldenhar syndrome, Oculoauicular Dysplasia, and Hemifacial Microsomia. Due to its complexity and inconsistent severity, most researchers consider Hemifacial Microsomia and Goldenhar syndrome as different aspects of OAVS, whereas a few others regard them as separate entities.[83]

OAVS encompasses a wide range of auditory atresias, anotias, and microtias, of which microtia is the most frequent. These congenital deformities may appear separate from, or as parts of, several other syndromes; for example, Alpert and velo-cardiofacial syndromes. Common ear deformities that may or may not be associated with this genetic defect are Blainville's, Stahl's, cup, and lop ear. The many OAVS characteristics that are found in other syndromes, like CHARGE and Treacher-Collins, further complicate classification.

## Frequency of Occurrence

OAVS's frequency of occurrence is variously estimated between 1 in 3,000 to 1 in 5,000 births. A 3:2 male over female predominance has been noted. Unilateral microtia is estimated to occur in 1 of 7,000 to 8,000 births. Bilateral forms have an estimated incidence of 1 in 20,000 births.[84] Among associated congenital malformations, facial clefts, and cardiac defects are the most common ones (each about 30% of infants with associated malformations).

Parents of OAVS children appear to have less than a 1-in-100 chance of bearing a second child with OAVS. Persons with OAVS have an estimated probability of about 3 in 100 of passing it on to their children.

Incidence data vary widely for microtia and anotia: European estimates range from fewer than 1 per 10,000 French births to over 2 per 10,000 Swedish births. A study of their epidemiology in Italy estimated their occurrences to be about 1.5 per 10,000 live births.[85] Another study estimates the occurrence of these defects between 1 in 7,000 to 10,000 live births.[86] In the United States, differences have been noted between racial and ethnic groups, with one estimate of 4 per 10,000 American Indian children.[87]

## Etiology

The cause(s) of these anomalies has yet to be determined with certainty. Some research suggests that they may be due to autosomal dominant inheritance, with variable expression and incomplete penetrance in an undetermined portion of cases.

OAVS has been classified as a spectrum disorder, rather than a syndrome. Environmental factors may be involved. For example, a rate of OAVS four times higher than in the general population has been found in children of Gulf War veterans.[88] A few cases have family histories that suggest inheritance of OAVS. With respect to microtia, fewer than 1 in 8 cases have a family history of ear anomalies. This rate suggests that, in most instances, the genetic basis for microtia is sporadic.

Another theory is that OAVS results from disruption of the blood supply during embryonic development, resulting in destruction of tissue in the first and second branchial arches that differentiates features of the face, skull, and ear. Yet another hypothesis notes that some teratogens, like thalidomide and accutane, have caused birth defects similar to those in OAVS.[89] These defects have also been found in some infants born to parents who survived the atomic bombing of Hiroshima. Multifactorial etiology comprised of some or all of the above has also been proposed as causal.[90]

In fully expressed OAVS, the microtic outer ear is usually accompanied by middle-ear abnormalities, including canal atresia and ossicular abnormalities. The middle-ear deformities range from diminished canal opening and minor ossicular abnormalities to fused, hypoplastic ossicles and failure of mastoid bone aeration.

Typically, OAVS includes anotia and/or microtia of the outer ears, narrow or absent external ear canals, and hearing impairment. The hearing loss may be conductive, sensorineural, or mixed. In a majority of cases, OAVS is bilateral, although its malformations may affect one side—usually the right side— more than the other.

## Diagnosis

When hypoplasia of the mandible or severe abnormality of the ears is apparent, these defects can be observed by ultrasound as early as the sixth to seventh weeks of embryologic development. If the facial asymmetry is not obvious, postgestational diagnosis may be delayed until the child reaches about 4 years of age.

These defects have been graded in accordance with the extent of their deviation from normal ears:

Grade I, a small ear with identifiable structures and smaller than normal external ear canal;

Grade II, partial outer ear with closed external ear canal;

Grade III, absence of the external ear and of the external ear canal and eardrum;

Grade IV, absence of the total ear or anotia.

The availability of CT and MRI technology provides the means of determining whether sensorineural structures are involved. Audiologic evaluation to determine the extent to which these malformations may cause hearing loss do not require special techniques beyond those usually applied in an audiologic examination.

## Management

OAVS arouses several potential medical and psychological concerns. Audiologic evaluation and evaluation of speech and language are essential to plan for management. Instituting early evaluation and treatment of hearing loss will reduce educational and speech-language delays.[91]

## *Surgery*

Surgery may be undertaken to correct the facial defects and to correct possible congenital heart defects. Lack of development of the upper and lower jaws can cause breathing and dental problems and interfere with feeding, defects that can be corrected surgically.[92,93]

Plastic and otologic surgery to reconstruct the ear and to correct problems in the middle ear usually requires multiple surgeries. To correct auricular defects, they are usually delayed until the affected child is 5 years of age, when it is expected that the auditory structures have attained the majority of their adult size.[94] If a fused malleus or stapedial fixation is present, a CT scan before attempting surgery may determine if the removal of the footplate will release a flood of perilymphatic fluid—a serious and possibly predictable complication.[95]

Much of the success of these operations depends on the artistic abilities of the surgeon. Another factor is the autogenous rib framework's resorption potential with subsequent loss of contour detail over time.[96]

## *Amplification*

If the cochlea and the auditory nVIII remain functional, patients with these anomalies may be able to hear with a bone-conduction aid. The BAHA (bone-anchored hearing aid) may be for others with OAVS (see Section 2.1).

## *Counseling*

Parent counseling is critical to overcome any guilt that parents of a child with this type of birth defect may feel (see also Section 2.3). Patients and their families may be referred to support groups that offer emotional support, companionship, and relevant information; for example, Hemifacial Microsomia/Goldenhar Syndrome Family Support Network,[97] Children's Craniofacial Association,[98] Atresia/Microtia Support Group,[99] Anophthalmia/Microphthalmia Registry[100] and Goldenhar Syndrome Support Network Society.[101]

## OSTEOGENESIS IMPERFECTA

Osteogenesis imperfecta (OI) is a congenital disease that affects collagen, a building block of bone. It has several synonyms and closely related conditions: Brittle Bone syndrome,

Bruck syndrome, Adair-Dighton syndrome, Van der Hoeve syndrome, Ekman-Lobstein syndrome—attesting to the diversity of its expressions.[102] A British otologist, first described OI in 1912, who noted cases of adult-onset deafness, blue sclerae, and brittle bones.[103]

## Frequency of Occurrence

OI has an estimated prevalence in the United States from 1 per 20,000 to 1 per 50,000 persons. Its worldwide prevalence is similarly rare. Race and gender do not appear to be factors in its occurrence, although substantial variations in prevalence have been noted in some samples taken in other countries. Because mild cases may go undiagnosed, it is possible that OI's prevalence has been underestimated.[104]

## Etiology

The causes of OI are indefinite. It generally has been classified as autosomal dominant, although no specific mutation has been identified as being responsible for it. An OI genetic defect can be inherited from a parent who carries the gene for OI, even if that parent does not manifest the disease.[105]

The onset of symptoms in OI varies, with bone fractures and hearing losses occurring at any developmental stage from prenatal to adulthood. The likelihood of a hearing loss increases with age, usually in adolescence or adulthood. About half of persons with OI have significant hearing losses, due to defects in the ossicles and inner ear.

The whites of the eyes of some patients with OI may have sclerae with a noticeably blue tint. All bones are weak in patients with OI, but the extent of brittleness differs from patient to patient. Those with Type 1 OI may be asymptomatic throughout their lives, although they are always at risk of fractures. Infants with Type 2 OI typically do not survive much past birth.

## Diagnosis

The diagnosis of OI requires collagen studies based on skin biopsies. The types of collagen dysfunction have been identified as Type I, mildest form; Type II, lethal form; Type III: progressive, severely deforming type; Type IV: moderately severe form, differentiated from Type 1 by white sclerae, and from Type III by autosomal dominant inheritance, and Type VII, moderately deforming condition found only among a small community of Native Americans.[106]

DNA testing of family members is recommended. Ultrasound and analyses of amniotic fluid enable diagnosis of severe OI in a fetus as young as 16 weeks postconception. OI may be diagnosed at birth if the condition is sufficiently severe.[107] Mild cases, however, may remain undetected, sometimes into adulthood, which may account for the possible underestimation of this disease.[108]

## Management

Management of OI concentrates on improving the patient's quality of life: amplification for any hearing loss, prompt repair of fractures, exercises to strength muscles, good nutrition, and similar measures.[109]

Bone-marrow transplants, transplants of mesenchymal stem cells, ingesting growth hormones, gene therapy to block the defective gene when the patient has one unaffected gene —all have been tried but none has been adopted for general practice.[110-113]

Genetic counseling should be provided all patients with OI and their families. Also, parents of a child with OI are sometimes accused of child abuse when they bring their child to an emergency room for treatment of broken bones.[114] The Osteogenesis Imperfecta Foundation can provide the support they may need in this and other circumstances.[115]

# PENDRED SYNDROME

Pendred syndrome (PS) comprises three features: congenital sensorineural hearing loss, enlargement of the thyroid gland (goiter), and positive perchlorate discharge. PS was described in 1896 by Vaughan Pendred, a British physician.

## Frequency of Occurrence

PS is among those now considered rare. In the period 1915 to 1922, in Switzerland, it occurred at a relatively high rate of 1.2 to 1.7 per 1,000 live births. By 1925, the rate of PS in that country decreased to 0.4 per 1,000—a rate considered applicable to most European countries.[116] The decrease was attributed to adding iodine to table salt, in order to prevent damage to the thyroid gland—a practice that is now common to landlocked areas that typically lack dietary iodine.

## Etiology

PS is an autosomal recessive trait that carries, among its components, the thyroid hormones that regulate cellular growth and metabolic rate. Research has established that the defective gene underlying PS is located on the long arm of chromosome 7.[117]

The congenital thyroid defect frequently causes a lag in intellectual development resulting in mental deficiency in addition to whatever effects are attributable to the sensorineural hearing loss. Deafness is present at birth, along with defective balance and malformation of a portion of the cochlea.

## Diagnosis

Early diagnosis is critical, as treating the goiter can slow the hearing loss and possibly prevent the onset of mental retardation. Landlocked areas of most countries now include iodine in the table salt, in order to limit the effects of a dysfunctional goiter.

## Management

Aside from treating the goiter deficiency, management for this syndrome focuses on treatment of the hearing loss, for which see Section 2.

# POMPE DISEASE

Pompe disease (PD) is a glycogen storage disease.[118] It was first described in 1977.[119] It is one of 49 known lysosomal-storage disorders.

## Frequency of Occurrence

PD is estimated to occur in 1 per 40,000 births in the United States. It probably affects between 50,000 and 100,000 people worldwide.

## Etiology

PD is inherited as an autosomal dominant trait that includes hearing loss in combination with hypoparathyroidism and renal dysplasia.[120]

A genetic mutation causes deficiency or lack of acid maltase. If this enzyme does not work properly, glycogen buildup in the cells damages principally the muscles. Researchers have identified 70 different mutations in the GAA gene that causes PD symptoms.

## Diagnosis

Diagnosis of PD is made by a skin biopsy or a blood test, although symptoms of extreme muscle weakness, especially in infants, alert clinicians to the disease.

The three forms of PD progress differently, depending on their onsets. Infants with PD usually show muscle weakness, such as trouble holding up their heads, in the first months postgestation. They usually die of heart failure and respiratory weakness before their first birthday. The childhood form progresses more slowly, but individuals with PD usually die before age 30 years. In the adult form, symptoms appear later and may be confused with multiple sclerosis.

Audiologic examinations of all patients with PD are indicated.[121] Some clinicians suspect middle- or inner-ear pathology rather than CNS involvement with cochlear pathology is the most likely cause of hearing loss in infantile PD.[122]

## Management

The U.S. Food and Drug Administration has approved Myozyme (alglucosidase alfa) for the treatment of PD. However, without enzyme replacement therapy, prognosis remains guarded and seems to depend on the age at onset.[123]

Diagnostic testing and genetic counseling are recommended for all family members of a patient with PD.

## Resources

Among the organizations to which patients and their families can turn for support and possible assistance are: Association for Glycogen Storage Disease,[124] Acid Maltase Deficiency Association,[125] and the Muscular Dystrophy Association.[126]

# TREACHER-COLLINS SYNDROME

Treacher-Collins syndrome (TCS) presents with distorted facial characteristics (Mandibulo-Facial Dysostosis) and hearing loss. TCS may also include cleft palate, atresia of the external canal, ossicular chain involvement, malformed or missing ears, outer corners of the eyes slanting down, coloboma of the lower eyelid, small lower jaw, unusually large mouth, large beaklike nose, small or obstructed nasal passages, and, occasionally, unusually small or missing thumbs.

## Frequency of Occurrence

TCS's incidence is estimated to be about 1 in 10,000 live births. The condition is named for the British ophthalmologist who first described it in 1900.

## Etiology

TCS results from a mutation of chromosome 5. This condition has variable expression, resulting in considerable variation in symptoms and severity from generation to generation. Based on an absence of TCS's occurrence in the family histories of patients with the disease, more than half of all cases are assumed to be new mutations. However, it is possible that the patients' parents carry the gene undetected, when manifestations of TCS are so mild as to go unnoticed.

## Diagnosis

Because of the variability in the underlying genetics, correctly diagnosing this condition can be difficult. A thorough family history and DNA analysis may be needed to resolve any doubts about its etiology in individual cases.

## Management

Defects that accompany TCS may be treated by surgery: tracheotomy to relieve the breathing difficulties, closing the coloboma to forestall eye infections, and correcting the cleft palate.

Children with TCS are usually intellectually average or above. After appropriate treatment—which includes prompt attention to their hearing losses—these children most often become normally functioning adults.

For advocacy and self-help groups, see the Treacher-Collins Foundation[127] and Children's Craniofacial Association.[128] The latter organization also has an interest in other similar physical anomalies.

## USHER SYNDROME (USH)

Ush consists of congenital hearing loss and progressive blindness due to retinitis pigmentosa. C. H. Usher, a British ophthalmologist, first identified this disorder in 1914.[129]

Refsum syndrome (Ref), also known as phytanic-acid-storage disease, is a related condition that shares the otic and ocular manifestations of Usher syndrome, but also includes cerebellar ataxia and chronic polyneuropathy.[130] Alstrom syndrome is another very rare genetically transmitted disorder that includes the dual sensory losses and other organ dysfunctions.[131] (See also Norrie disease.)

### Frequency of Occurrence

Usher syndrome accounts for about half the prevalence of deafblindness in the United States. Its prevalence in the population is estimated to be approximately 3 per 100,000 on average.[132,133] The associated Ref syndrome is rare and, in some instances, affected persons' condition may be attributed, incorrectly, to Ush.[134]

### Etiology

Ush and Ref are autosomal recessive syndromes. Ush can be subdivided into three types on the basis of clinical findings: Type I, both hearing, visual, and vestibular impairments; Type II, hearing and visual impairments without vestibular impairment; Type III, variable amounts of vestibular impairment accompanying the twin sensory defects.[135]

### Diagnosis

The hearing loss varies from moderate to profound. Its onset is congenital,[136] and it is usually progressive, the increase probably due to exogenous rather than endogenous factors.

The visual impairment usually becomes manifest in adolescence, with night blindness its first symptom. However, ophthalmologists can detect retinitis pigmentosa in a 6-year-old child. An electroretinograph can detect the condition even if it is not obvious to the ophthalmoscope. The visual loss worsens idiosyncratically, ending in blindness usually after the third or forth decade. A new test, the USMChip, analyzes for all eight optic variations of Ush. It can be obtained from the National Center for the Study and Treatment of Usher Syndrome.[137]

The differential diagnosis between Ush and Ref can be made clinically, in that Ref's symptoms have an onset from late childhood to early adulthood. DNA analysis and hematologic analyses can confirm the diagnosis.

## Management

Once Ush is diagnosed, a question may arise: When should children with Ush be told of its future consequences? The earlier individuals with Ush begin preparations for deafblindness, the more likely their preparations will be successful.[138] The fear that telling children they have Ush will damage them emotionally is belied by experience: young children overcome the emotional impact of the diagnosis more readily than older ones or adults and they can begin developing needed skills and making long-term career choices that will be compatible with their futures.

Despite the difficulties that deafblindness imposes on communication, the needs for information and emotional support remain. Counseling patients with Ush should, therefore, not be avoided.[139,140] For information and assistance, contact the Helen Keller National Center for Deaf-Blind Youth and Adults, Sands Point, New York, via E-mail at HKNCinfo@hknc.org

## VESTIBULAR AQUEDUCT AND SEMICIRCULAR CANAL MALFORMATIONS (VASCM)

VASCM consists of malformations of the vestibular portions of the inner ear. The condition is associated with early-onset sensorineural hearing loss.

## Frequency of Occurrence

Although VASCMs are thought to be rare, they may be under-reported because those with relatively mild or absent symptoms are probably undiagnosed.

## Etiology

Familial cases of VASCM have been reported, which suggests autosomal dominant inheritance. However, recessive inheritance has also been postulated.

The inner-ear malformations are usually bilateral, and the resulting effects may be progressive. They often include vestibular symptoms, such as, vertigo and poor muscular coordination. Cochlear and semicircular canal deformities may also accompany VASCM. As the formation of the semicircular canals begins in the sixth gestational week, mutations are most likely to occur in that period.

## Diagnosis

Isolated lateral canal defects are the most commonly identified VASCM seen on temporal-bone imaging studies.

Following an audiometric examination that measures the extent of the hearing loss, radiologic and MRIs may also aid in detecting VASCM.

## Management

Providing prompt amplification is the treatment of choice for VASCM. Because progressive hearing losses probably result from hydrodynamic effects and possibly from disruption of the labyrinthine membrane, regular audiologic monitoring is essential to adjust amplification in accordance with anticipated changes. If amplification fails to yield good results, a cochlear implant should be considered.

# VELOCARDIOFACIAL SYNDROME (VCFS)

VCFS has multiple features, of which the most common are cleft palate, cardiac defects, and a distinctive facial appearance (long face, almond-shaped eyes, wide nose, and small ears). A speech-language pathologist first described this condition, in 1978, so it is also known as Shprintzen syndrome. Because of the wide variety in its expression, it has further been named DiGeorge, Sedlaãková, and Cayler syndromes.[141]

## Frequency of Occurrence

Researchers consider VCFS to be the most common contiguous-gene-deletion syndrome in humans and one of the most common syndromes including congenital heart disease.[142]

VCFS adds a relatively small amount to the prevalence of hearing disorders, as congenital hearing losses occur in a minority of persons with VCFS. However, the structure of their auditory canals makes them susceptible to otitis media, which, in turn, may lead to serous otitis media and potentially to conductive hearing loss. Although in VCFS the hearing loss is typically conductive, resulting from the distortion of the bony structure that houses the ear, the hearing loss may become sensorineural if the cochlea is compromised.

Approximately 5 to 8% of children with cleft palates also have some additional VCFS characteristics, which may or may not include hearing loss. One parent with VCFS has a 50% likelihood of having a child with some or all of the VCFS features.[143]

## Etiology

VCFS occurs sporadically. Although it is generally regarded as being genetic and having autosomal dominant transmission, in only a minority of instances has its specific inheritance been established.

The reason for the wide variety of phenotypes associated with VCFS remains open: Is the broad spectrum of anomalies the result of a single gene, by most or all of some deleted genes, or by an interaction between the genes in the deleted region and the other genes in the genome? Each of these hypotheses has had support, but none has achieved consensus.

## Diagnosis

The presenting symptoms are highly variable because VCFS is often the trigger for a number of developmental malformation sequences and because its causes appear to be complex. The lack of understanding of its etiology may be due in part to its rarity, the variability in its manifestations, and a lack of focus by clinicians on the few cases they encounter.

## Management

Aside from correcting the cleft palate, attention should be directed to the hearing loss, which should be treated promptly. Annual audiologic evaluation to determine the onset of acquired hearing loss should be a management requirement.

# WAARDENBURG SYNDROME (WAAS)

WaaS consists of mild to profound sensorineural hearing loss and pigmentary features: most prominently a patch of white scalp hair and heterochromic irises. The complete expression comprises additional physical anomalies that include lateral displacement of the medial canthi of the eyelids and hyperpigmentation of the skin.

A Dutch physician at St. Michielsgestel Institut voor Doven, a school for deaf students in the Netherlands, first noted its auditory-pigmentary features.[144]

## Frequency of Occurrence

WaaS is the most common of the auditory-pigmentary syndromes that experts estimate affect about half of persons with dominant, syndromic hearing loss. Estimates of the incidence of this syndrome center about 1 per 4,000 live births. About 3% of congenital deafness has been attributed to it and its various expressions, although these estimates vary from place to place, over time.

For years it was assumed that the syndrome was limited to Dutch children, but this has since proved incorrect, with WAAS appearing worldwide. The belief that the syndrome did not occur among non-white persons has also proved to be wrong, having been noted among Chinese, Japanese, Maoris, Asian Indians, and other ethnic and racial groups.[145]

## Etiology

WaaS is transmitted as an autosomal dominant trait.[146] When partial expressions occur, suggesting incomplete penetrance, inquiry should be made about all family members, in order to detect those with incipient indicators. For example, a child with sensorineural deafness but no other features of WaaS may have a normally hearing father who displays only heterochromatic irises and a grandfather who had heterochromatic irises and a white forelock or afterlock. Neither of these parents may have had a hearing loss, but such a family history would indicate the likelihood that the offspring with the hearing loss has a variant of WaaS.

Four types have been identified: WaaS Types I and II include lateral displacement of the inner canthus of each eye, pigmentary abnormalities of hair, iris, and skin, and sensorineural deafness. When WaaS Types I and II combine with upper-limb abnormalities, the result is WaaS Type III or Klein-Waardenburg syndrome.[147] When WaaS Types I and II occur with Hirschsprung disease, the result is labeled WaaS Type IV, Waardenburg-Shah syndrome.[148]

## Diagnosis

The physical characteristics of WaaS make a diagnosis fairly obvious in a fully expressed case: in addition to the deafness, the heterochromia and facial anomalies usually suffice. In instances of incomplete penetrance and partial expression, the diagnosis often depends on obtaining a thorough family history and DNA analysis.

## Management

There is no particular management that is unique to this syndrome. However, genetic counseling should be made available to prospective parents to determine if they carry the abnormal gene.

# WILDERVANCK SYNDROME (WILS)

WilS, also known as Cervico-Oculo-Acoustic syndrome, consists of profound congenital deafness, Klippel-Feil malformation of the spine (shortness of the neck due to reduction in the number of cervical vertebrae and low hairline) and Duane syndrome (abducens paralysis of one or both eyes). It may include cleft palate, spina bifida, torticollis, and split hands and feet.[149]

## Frequency of Occurrence

WilS is a rare genetic disorder that primarily affects females. The female-to-male ratio is estimated to be 10:1, and the incidence of deafness in females is estimated to be about 1 to 2%.[150] The sex ratio is attributed to partial limitation of a mutant allele resulting in an excess of females.

## Etiology

The mode of inheritance remains undetermined. One hypothesis attributes inheritance to autosomal dominance with incomplete penetrance and variable expressivity,[151] although another expert describes its inheritance as non-Mendelian.[130] There are no reported examples of multiple cases in a family. Another study suggests it is due to polygenic inheritance with limitation to females and lethality for males.[152]

## Diagnosis

It may be that this condition occurs with greater frequency than has been reported because its expressive variability makes diagnosis uncertain. However, the full expression of WilS leaves no doubt of its presence.

## Management

There is no specific therapy for this condition. However, early treatment of the hearing disorder is essential to avoid speech and language delays that usually accompany congenital hearing loss.[153]

# X-LINKED INHERITANCE

There are no other aspects of the X-linked inheritance of hearing loss that distinguish it—that is, no other symptoms typically accompany the hearing loss—hence, it is nonsyndromic. However, a number of syndromes also appear to be X-linked, and their discussion is inserted where appropriate in the relevant discussions (as an example, see Norrie disease).

## Frequency of Occurrence

Nonsyndromic X-linked deafness is relatively uncommon, typically reported at rates considerably lower than 1 per 2,000 live births.

## Etiology

The genes causing these types of inherited deafness rest on the X chromosome. All sons and none of the daughters in a family with X-linked deafness will have hearing losses. None of the fathers with hearing losses will have affected sons with genetic hearing loss because males have only one X chromosome, which they inherit from their mothers. When the mother has the gene, each of her sons will have a 50/50 chance of inheriting the X-linked gene and subsequent hearing loss. All daughters of affected fathers will be carriers, because they inherit their father's single X chromosome. But they will not have a hearing loss from that cause themselves. As carriers, however, they will pass along the mutation.

A person with X-linked hearing loss due to mutations of a gene on the X chromosome will likely have a fixed stapes footplate that produces a conductive component to the hearing loss. Congenital conductive hearing loss is often associated with middle-ear fluid, but it can also be due to ossicular-chain abnormalities; for example, fused malleus or stapedial fixation. The hearing loss might also arise from inner-ear malformations, such as Mondini aplasia and Scheibe aplasia. These malformations may appear with heritable conditions, like Waardenburg and Pendred syndromes, and may occur unilaterally or bilaterally. They are associated with both conductive and sensorineural hearing losses.

## Diagnosis

Family history, DNA analysis, and CT scan—to identify the ossicular chain disorder, if any—provide the principal bases for diagnosis.

## Management

Middle-ear anomalies are treated surgically, and when successful, usually results in a restoration of hearing lost due to a defective conductive component. If surgery is either infeasible or unsuccessful, amplification and speech and hearing therapies provide useful options. Any conductive components should be identified and treated early, in order to prevent speech and language retardation.

# REFERENCES

1. Gelfand SA, ed. *Essentials of Audiology*. 2nd ed. New York, NY: Thieme, 2001.

2. Devarajan P. Alport syndrome. Retrieved December 2006 from http://www.emedicine.com/ped/topic74.htm

3. Information on Alport syndrome. Retrieved September 2007 from http://www.boystownhospital.org/hearing/info/genetics/syndromes/ Alport.asp

4. Barker DF, Pruchno CJ, Jiang K, et al. A mutation causing Alport syndrome with tardive hearing loss is common in the western United States. *Am J Hum Genet*. 1996;58(6): 1157-1165.

5. Eckstein JD, Filip DJ, Watts JC. Hereditary thrombocytopenia, deafness and renal disease. *Ann Internal Med*. 1975;82: 639-645.

6. Epstein CJ, Sahud MA, Piel CF, et al. Hereditary macrothrombocytopathia, nephritis and deafness. *Am J Med*. 1972;52: 299-310.

7. Saxena R. Alport syndrome. Retrieved 2007 from http://www.emedicine.com/med/topic110.htm

8. Musiek FE, Weider DJ, Mueller RJ. Audiologic findings in Charcot-Marie-Tooth disease. *Arch Otolaryngol*. 1982;108: 595-599.

9. Charcot-Marie-Tooth syndrome. Retrieved April 2007 from http://www.emedicine.com/orthoped/topic43.htm

10. Nance WE, Kearsey MJ. Relevance of connexin deafness (DFNB1) to human evolution. *Am J Hum Genet*. 2004;74(6): 1081-1087.

11. Hamiel OP, Raas-Rothschild A, Upadhyaya M, et al. Hereditary motor-sensory neuropathy (Charcot-Marie-Tooth disease) with nerve deafness: a new variant. *J Pediatr*. 1993;123: 431-434.

12. Kovach MJ, Lin J, Boyadjiev S, et al. A unique point mutation in the PMP22 gene is associated with Charcot-Marie-Tooth disease and deafness. *Am J Hum Genet*. 1999;64:1580-1593.

13. Charcot-Marie-Tooth disease. Retrieved February 2007 from http://www.ncbi.nlm.nih.gov/books

14. Charcot-Marie-Tooth Association. Retrieved 2007 from http://www.charcot-marie-tooth.org

15. Alpert syndrome. Retrieved October 2007 from http://www. biology-online.org/dictionary/alpert_syndrome

16. Online Mendelian Inheritance in Man. Accessed at http:// www.ncbi.nlm.nih.gov/omim

17. Lee KJ. *Essential Otolaryngology*. 4th ed. New York, NY: Medical Examination Publishing Company; 1987.

18. Anderson PJ, Cox TC, Roscioli T, et al. Somatic FGFR and TWIST mutations are not a common cause of isolated non-syndromic single suture craniosynostosis. *J Craniofac Surg.* 2007;18(2):312–314.

19. Kaplan LC. Clinical assessment and multispecialty management of Alpert syndrome. *Clin Plast Surg.* 1991;18(2):1–9.

20. Friedman E, Blau A, Farfel Z. A variant of the "DIDMOAD" syndrome (diabetes insipidus, diabetes mellitus, optic atrophy and deafness). *Clin Genet.* 1986;29:79–82.

21. Cremers, C, Wijdeveld P, Pinckers A. Juvenile diabetes mellitus, optic atrophy, hearing loss, diabetes insipidus, atonia of the urinary tract and bladder, and other abnormalities (Wolfram syndrome): a review of 88 cases from the literature with personal observations on 3 new patients. *Acta Paediatr Scand.* 1977;264(suppl):3–16.

22. Wolfram DJ, Wagener HP. Diabetes mellitus and simple optic atrophy among siblings: report of four cases. *Mayo Clinic Proc.* 1938;13:715–718.

23. Khanim F, Kirk J, Latif F, et al. WFS1/Wolframin mutations, Wolfram syndrome, and associated diseases. *Hum Mutat.* 2001;17:357–367.

24. Eiberg H, Hansen L, Kjer, et al. Autosomal dominant optic atrophy associated with hearing impairment and impaired glucose regulation caused by a missense mutation in the WFS1 gene. *J Med Genet.* 2006;43:435–440.

25. Strom TM, Hortnagel K, Hofmann S, et al. Diabetes insipidus, diabetes mellitus, optic atrophy and deafness (DIDMOAD) caused by mutations in a novel gene (wolframin) coding for a predicted transmembrane protein. *Hum Molec Genet.* 1998;7:2021–2028.

26. Lesperance MM, Hall JW, San Augustin TB, et al. Mutations in the Wolfram syndrome Type 1 gene (WFS1) define a clinical entity of dominant sensorineural hearing loss. *Arch Otolaryngol Head Neck Surg.* 2003;129(4):411–420.

27. Vaughan N, James K, McDermott D, et al. A five-year prospective study of diabetes and hearing loss in a veteran population. *Otol Neurotol*. 2005;27(1):37–43.

28. Smith RJH, Huygen PLM. Making sense of nonsyndromic deafness. *Arch Otolaryngol Head Neck Surg*. 2003;129: 405–406.

29. Worldwide Society of Families Living with Wolfram Syndrome. Retrieved December 2006 from http://www.wolfram syndrome.org/

30. Maroteaux P, Lamy M. La pseudo-polydystrophie de Hurler. *La Presse Medicale*. 1966;74:2889–2892.

31. Hurler G. Uber einen Typ multipler Abartungen, vorwiegend am Skelettsystem. *Zeitschrift fur Kinderheilkunde*. 1919;24: 220–234.

32. Hunter CA. A rare disease in two brothers. *Proc Roy Soc Med*. 1917;10:6–7.

33. National Institute of Neurological Diseases and Stroke. *Mucolipidoses Fact Sheet*. Publication No. 03-5115. Bethesda, Md: Office of Communications and Public Liaison; February 13, 2007.

34. Staba SL, Escolar ML, Poe M, et al. Cord-blood transplants from unrelated donors in patients with Hurler's syndrome. *N Engl J Med*. 2004;350(19):1960–1969.

35. Therapy for Hurler disease. Retrieved May 2006 from http://www.nlm.nih.gov/medlineplus/ency/article/001203

36. Asif A, Christie PT, Grigorieva IV, et al. Functional characterization of GATA3 mutations causing the hypoparathyroidism-deafness-renal (HDR) dysplasia syndrome: insight into mechanisms of DNA binding by the GATA3 transcription factor. *Hum Molec Gene*. 2007;16(3):265–275.

37. Ali A, Christie PT, Grigorieva IV, et al. Functional characterisation of GATA3 mutations causing the Hypoparathyroidism-Deafness-Renal Dysplasia (HDR) syndrome: insight into mechanisms of DNA binding by the GATA3 transcription factor. Retrieved January 2007 from Human Molecular Genetics Advance Access doi:10.1093/hmg/ddl454

38. Nesbit MA, Bowl MR, Harding B, et al. Characterization of GATA3 mutations in the hypoparathyroidism, deafness, and renal dysplasia (HDR) syndrome. *J Bio Chem*. 2004;279: 22624–22634.

39. Van Looija MAJ, Meijers-Heijboerb H, Beetzc R, et al. Characteristics of hearing loss in HDR (hypoparathyroidism, sensorineural deafness, renal dysplasia) syndrome. *Audiol Otol.* 2006;11:373–379.

40. Jervell A, Lange-Nielsen F. Congenital deaf-mutism, functional heart disease with prolongation of Q-T interval and sudden death. *Am Heart J.* 1957;54:59–68.

41. Lehmann MH, Timothy KW, Frankovich D, et al. Age-gender influence on the rate-corrected QT interval and the QT-heart rate relation in families with genotypically characterized long QT syndrome. *J Am Coll Cardiol.* 1997;29(1):93–99.

42. Neyroud N, Tesson F, Denjoy I, et al. A novel mutation in the potassium channel gene KVLQT1 causes the Jervell and Lange-Nielsen cardio-auditory syndrome. *Nature Genet.* 1997;15:186–189.

43. Schultze-Bahr E, Haverkamp W, Wedekind H et al. Autosomal recessive long-QT syndrome (Jervell Lange-Nielsen) is genetically heterogeneous. *Hum Genet.* 1997;100(5–6):573–576.

44. Splawski I, Timothy K, Vincent GM, et al. Molecular basis of the long QT syndrome associated with deafness. *N Engl J Med.* 1997;336:1562–1567.

45. Kartagener M. Zur pathogenese der Bronchiectasien. Mitteilung bronchiectasien bei situs viscerum inversus. *Betrage Klinikus Tuberkennis.* 1933;83:498–501.

46. Afzelius BA. A human syndrome caused by immotile cilia. *Science.* 1976;193(4250):317–319.

47. Chin GY, Karas DE, Kashgarian M. Correlation of presentation and pathologic condition in primary ciliary dyskinesia. *Arch Otolaryngol Head Neck Surg.* 2002;128(11):1292–1294.

48. Ruben RJ. The pediatric otolaryngologic assessment of the child with suspected hearing loss. In: Gerber SE, ed. *The Handbook of Pediatric Audiology.* Washington, DC: Gallaudet University Press; 1996.

49. Teknos TN, Metson R, Chasse T. New developments in the diagnosis of Kartagener's syndrome. *Otolaryngol Head Neck Surg.* 1997;116(1):68–74.

50. United Mitochondrial Disease Foundation. Retrieved May 2007 from http://www.umdf.org

51. El-Schahawi M, Lopez de Munain A, Sarrazin AM, et al. Two large Spanish pedigrees with nonsyndromic sensorineural deaf-

ness and the mtDNA mutation at nt 1555 in the 12s rRNA gene: evidence of heteroplasmy. *Neurology.* 1997;48:453–456.

52. Guan M-X. Prevalence of mitochondrial 12S rRNA mutations associated with aminoglycoside ototoxicity. *Volta Rev.* 2005; 105(3):211–227.

53. Hutchins TP, Cortopassi GA. Mitochondria and risk for deafness. *Am J Audiol.* 1995;4:12–14.

54. Merchant SN, McKenna MJ, Nadol JB, et al. Temporal bone histopathologic and genetic studies in Mohr-Tranebjaerg syndrome (DFN-1). *Otol Neurotol.* 2001;22:506–511.

55. Mohr J, Mageroy K. Sex-linked deafness of a possibly new type. *Acta Genet Statistic Med.* 1960;10:54–62.

56. Tranebjaerg L, Hamel BCJ, Gabreels FJM, et al. A de novo missense mutation in a critical domain of the X-linked DDP gene causes the typical deafness-dystonia-optic atrophy syndrome. *Eur J Hum Genet.* 2000;8:464–467.

57. Orphanet Journal of Rare Diseases. Retrieved May 2007 from http://www.ojrd.com

58. Rutter J, Probst B, McKnight SL. Coordinate regulation of sugar flux and translation by PAS kinase. *Cell.* 2002;111(1): 17–28.

59. Koehler CM, Leuenberger D, Merchant S, et al. Human deafness dystonia syndrome is a mitochondrial disease. *Proc Nat Acad Sci.* 1999;96: 2141–2146.

60. Roesch K, Hynds PJ, Varga R, et al. The calcium-binding aspartate/glutamate carriers, citrin and aralar1, are new substrates for the DDP1/TIMM8a-TIMM13 complex. *Hum Molec Genet.* 2004;13: 2101–2111.

61. Bahmad F, Merchant SM, Nadol JB, et al. Otopathology in Mohr-Tranebjaerg syndrome. *Laryngoscope.* 2007;117:1202–1208.

62. Tranebjaerg L, Schwartz C, Eriksen H, et al. A new X-linked recessive deafness syndrome with blindness, dystonia, fractures, and mental deficiency is linked to Xq22. *J Med Genet.* 1995;32:257–263.

63. Yamasoba T, Tsukuda K, Oka Y, et al. Cochlear histopathology associated with mitochondrial transfer of RNALeu (UUR) gene mutation. *Neurology.* 1999;52:1705–1707.

64. Ciafaloni E, Ricci E, Shanske S, et al. MELAS: Clinical features, biochemistry, and molecular genetics. *Ann Neurol.* 1992; 31(4):391–398.

65. Sue CM, Bruno C, Andreu AL, et al. Infantile encephalopathy associated with the MELAS A3243G mutation. *J Pediatr*. 1999;134(6).696-700.

66. Feigenbaum, A, Chitayat, D, Robinson B, et al. The expanding clinical phenotype of the tRNA (Leu(UUR)) A + G mutation. *J Med Genet*. 1996;62:398-403.

67. Hesterlee S. Mitochondrial myopathy: an energy crisis in the cells. *Quest*. 1999;6(4):1-17.

68. Thambisetty M, Newman NJ, Glass JD, et al. A practical approach to the diagnosis and management of MELAS: case report and review. *Neurologist*. 2002;8(5):302-312.

69. Pikus AT. Profile in Type 1 and 2 neurofribromatosis. *J Am Acad Audiol*. 1995;6(1):54-62.

70. Barker DF, Wright E, Nguyen K, et al. Gene for von Recklinghausen neurofibromatosis is in the pericentromeric region of chromosome 17. *Science*. 1987;236(4805):1100-1102.

71. Rouleau GA, Wetelecki W, Haines JL, et al. Genetic linkage of bilateral acoustic neurofibromatosis to a DNA marker on chromosome 22. *Nature*. 1987;329(6136):246-248.

72. Parry DM, Eldridge R, Kaiser-Kupfer MI, et al. Neurofibromatosis 2 (NF2): clinical characteristics of 63 affected individuals and clinical evidence for heterogeneity. *Am J Med Genet*. 1994;52(4):450-461.

73. Forstman BJ, Kuszyk BS, Urban BA, et al. Neurofibromatosis Type 1: a diagnostic mimicker at CT. *Radiographics*. 2001; 21(3):601-612.

74. DeBella K, Szudek J, Friedman JM. Use of the National Institutes of Health criteria for diagnosis of neurofibromatosis 1 in children. *Pediatrics*. 2000;105(3, pt 1):608-614.

75. Latoo M, Mohammed L, Ahmed R, et al. Neurofibromatosis type 2 (NF2): a rare cause of teenage deafness. *JK-Practitioner*. 2006:13(1):39-40.

76. See Section 2.2.

77. Howell SJ, Wilton P, Lindberg A, et al. Growth hormone replacement and the risk of malignancy in children with neurofibromatosis. *J Pediatr*. 1998;113(2):210-205.

78. Liebermann F, Korf BR. Emerging approaches toward the treatment of neurofibromatosis. *Genet Med*. 1999;1(4):158-164.

79. Neurofibromatosis, Inc. Retrieved September 2007 from http://www.nfinc.org

80. Acoustic Neuroma Foundation. Retrieved May 2007 from http://www.anausa.org

81. Riccardi, V.M., Eichner, J.E. *Neurofibromatosis: Phenotype, Natural History, and Pathogenesis*. Baltimore, Md: Johns Hopkins University Press; 1986.

82. Norrie Disease Association. Retrieved May 2007 from http://www.helix.mgh.harvard.edu

83. Scholtz AW, Fish JH. Kammen-Jolly K, et al. Goldenhar's syndrome: congenital hearing deficit of conductive or sensorineural origin? Temporal bone histopathologic study. *Otol Neurotol*. 2001;22(4):501-505.

84. Baur B. Reconstruction of microtia and acquired auricular defects. In: Mustarde JC, Jackson I, eds. *Plastic Surgery in Infancy and Childhood*. London, UK: Churchill Livingston; 1988.

85. Mastroiacovo P, Corchia C, Botto LD, et al. Epidemiology and genetics of microtia-anotia: a registry based study on over one million births. *J Med Genet*. 1995;32:453-457.

86. Harris J, Kallen HJ, Robert E. The epidemiology of anotia and microtia. *J Med Genet*. 1996;33(10):809-813.

87. Jaffe B. The incidence of ear diseases in the Navajo Indians. *Laryngoscope*. 1968;79:2126-2134.

88. Gulf War babies. Retrieved April 2007 from http://www.widesmiles.org/syndrom/hmsgold/gulfwar.html

89. Davidson J, Hyde ML, Alberti PW. Epidemiologic patterns in childhood hearing loss: a review. *Int J Pediatr Otorhinolaryngol*. 1989;17(3):239-266.

90. Gupta A, Patton MA. Familial microtia with meatal atresia and conductive deafness in five generations. *Am J Med Genet*. 1995;59(2):238-241.

91. Linstrom CJ, Aziz MH, Romo T. Unilateral aural atresia in childhood: case selection and rehabilitation. *J Otolaryngol*. 1995;24(3):168-179.

92. Romo T, Presti PM, Yalamanchili HR. Medpor alternative for microtia repair. *Fac Plast Surg Clin North Am*. 2006;14(2):129-136.

93. Romo T, Fozo MS, Sclafani AP. Microtia reconstruction using a porous polyethylene framework. *Fac Plast Surg*. 2000;16(1):15-22.

94. Tanzer RC. Microtia: A long-term follow-up of 44 reconstructed auricles. *Plast Reconst Surg*. 1999;104:319-335.

95. Congenital aural atresia. Retrieved October 2007 from http://www.bcm.edu/oto/grand/11295.html

96. Brent B. Technical advances in ear reconstruction and autogenous rib cartilage grafts: personal experience with 1,200 cases. *Plast Recons Surg.* 1999;164:319-335.

97. Hemifacial Microsomia/Goldenhar Syndrome Family Support Network. Retrieved May 2007 from http://www.widesmiles.org/syndrom/hmsgold

98. Children's Craniofacial Association. Retrieved May 2007 from http://www.ccakids.com

99. Atresia/Microtia Support Group. Retrieved May 2007 from http://www.atresiamicrotia-subscribe @yahoo groups.com

100. Anophthalmia/ Microphthalmia Registry. Retrieved July 2007 from http://www.angelfire.com/mi/microphthalmia

101. Goldenhar Syndrome Support Network Society. Retrieved July 2007 from http://www.goldenhar syndrome.org

102. Plotkin H, Primorac D, Rowe D. Osteogenesis imperfecta. In: Glorieux F, Pettifor J, Juppner J, eds. *Pediatric Bone: Biology and Disease.* Boston, Mass: Academic Press; 2003:314-451.

103. Rauch F, Glorieux FH. Osteogenesis imperfecta. *Lancet.* 2004;24:363(9418):1377-1385.

104. Plotkin H. Syndromes with congenital brittle bones. *BMC Pediatr.* 2004;4(16):1471-2431.

105. Plotkin H. Two questions about osteogenesis imperfecta. *J Pediatr Orthoped.* 2006;26:148-149.

106. Plotkin H, Lutz R. Osteoporosis in pediatrics. In: Deng HW, Liu Y, eds. *Current Topics in Osteoporosis.* New York, NY: World Scientific; 2005.

107. Rauch F, Travers R, Parfitt AM, et al. Static and dynamic bone hystomorphometry in children with osteogenesis imperfecta. *Bone.* 2000;26: 581-589.

108. Plotkin H, Lutz R. Osteoporosis in pediatrics. In: Deng HW, Liu Y, eds. *Current Topics in Osteoporosis.* New York, NY: World Scientific; 2005.

109. Esposito P, Turman K, Scherl S, et al. Percutaneous surgical treatment of multiple lower extremity deformities in children with osteogenesis imperfecta. In: *Proceedings of 2006 Annual Meeting of the Pediatric Orthopaedic Society of North America.* Rosemont, Ill: Pediatric Orthopaedic Society of North America; 2006.

110. Niyibizi C, Wang S, Mi Z, et al. Gene therapy approaches for osteogenesis imperfecta. *Gene Ther*. 2004;11(4):408–416.

111. Rauch F, Glorieux FH. Osteogenesis imperfecta. *Lancet*. 2004;24:363:1377–1385.

112. Sakkers R, Kok D, Engelbert R, et al. Skeletal effects and functional outcome with olpadronate in children with osteogenesis imperfecta: a two-year randomised placebo-controlled study. *Lancet*. 2004;363(9419):1427–1431.

113. Rauch F, Munns C, Land C et al. Pamidronate in children and adolescents with osteogenesis imperfecta: effect of treatment discontinuation. *J Clin Endocrin Metabol*. 2006;91: 1268–1274.

114. Child Abuse Allegations (vs. Osteogenesis Imperfecta). Retrieved February 2000 from http://www.oif.org

115. Ontogenesis Imperfecta Foundation. Access at http://www.oif.org

116. Trotter WR. The association of deafness with thyroid dysfunction. *Br Med J*. 1960;16:19–28.

117. Coyle B, Coffey R, Armour JAL, et al. Pendred syndrome (goiter and sensorineural hearing loss) maps to chromosome 7 in the region containing the nonsyndromic deafness gene DFNB4. *Nature Genet*. 1996;12:421–423.

118. Muroya K, Hasegawa T, Ito Y, et al. GATA3 abnormalities and the phenotypic spectrum of HDR syndrome. *J Med Genet*. 2001;38:374–380.

119. Barakat AY, D'Albora JB, Martin MM, et al. Familial nephrosis, nerve deafness, and hypoparathyroidism. *J Pediatr*. 1977;91: 61–64.

120. Bilous RW, Murty G, Parkinson DB, et al. Brief report: autosomal dominant familial hypoparathyroidism, sensorineural deafness, and renal dysplasia. *N Engl J Med*. 1992;327:1069–1074.

121. Van der Wees J, van Looij MAJ, de Ruiter MM, et al. Hearing loss following GATA3 haploinsufficiency is caused by cochlear disorder. *Neurobiol Dis*. 2004;16:169–178.

122. Kamphoven JH, de Ruiter MM, Winkel LP, et al. Hearing loss in infantile Pompe's disease and determination of underlying pathology in the knockout mouse. *Neurobiol Dis*. 2004; 16:14–20.

123. Van den Hout JMP, Kamphoven JHJ, Winkel LPF, et al. Long-term intravenous treatment of Pompe disease with recombinant

human α-glucosidase from milk. *Pediatrics*. 2004;113(5): 448–457.

124. Association for Glycogen Storage Disease. Retrieved February 2007 from http://www.agsdus.org

125. Acid Maltase Deficiency Association. Retrieved May 2007 from http://www.amda-pompe.org

126. Muscular Dystrophy Association. Retrieved July 2007 from http://www.mda.org

127. Treacher Collins Foundation. Retrieved May 2007 from http://www.treachercollinsfnd.org

128. Children's Craniofacial Association. Retrieved January 2007 from http://www.ccakids.com

129. Usher CH. On the inheritance of retinitis pigmentosa, with notes of cases. *Royal London Ophthalmol Hosp Rep*. 1914; 19:130.

130. Horoupian D. Pathology of the central auditory pathways and cochlear nerve. In: Alberti PW, Ruben RJ, eds. *Otologic Medicine and Surgery*. New York, NY: Churchill Livingstone; 1988.

131. Welsh LW. Alstom syndrome: progressive deafness and blindness. *Ann Otol Rhinol Laryngol*. 2007;116(4):281–285.

132. Hicks WM, Hicks DE. The Usher's syndrome adolescent: programming implications for school administrators, teachers, and residential advisors. In: Huebner HM, Prickett JG, Welch TR, et al, eds. *Hand in Hand: Selected Reprints and Annotated Bibliography on Working with Students Who Are Deaf-Blind*. New York, NY: American Foundation for the Blind Press; 1995.

133. Wolf EG, Delk MT, Schein JD. *Needs Assessment of Services to Deaf-Blind Individuals*. Washington, DC: Rehabilitation and Education Experts (REDEX) Inc; 1982.

134. Refsum disease. Retrieved April 2007 from http://www.bchealthguide.org/kbase/nord/nord348.htm

135. Kirchner C. *Data on Blindness and Visual Impairment in the U.S: A Resource Manual on Characteristics, Education, Employment and Service Delivery*. New York, NY: American Foundation for the Blind; 1985.

136. Lustig LR, Niparko JK. Sensorineural hearing loss. In: Lustig LR, Niparko JK, eds. *Clinical Neurotology*. London, UK: Martin Dunitz; 2002:161–174.

137. Kimber L. Usher syndrome. Retrieved August 2006 from http://www.girlsandboystown.org/home.asp

138. Michael MG, Paul PV. Early intervention for infants with deafblindness. In: Huebner HM, Prickett JG, Welch TR, Joffee E, eds. *Hand in Hand: Selected Reprints and Annotated Bibliography on Working with Students Who Are Deaf-Blind.* New York, NY: American Foundation for the Blind Press; 1995.

139. Ingraham CL, Vernon M, Clemente B, et al. Sex education for deaf-blind youths and adults. *J Vis Imp Blind.* 2000;94: 741-745.

140. Ingraham C.L., Vernon M. Mental health counseling with deafblind students: recommendations for families and professionals. In: Ingraham CL, ed. *Transition Planning for Students Who Are DeafBlind.* Knoxville, Tenn: PEPNet-South; 2007:1-15.

141. Shprintzen RJ. Velo-cardio-facial syndrome: a distinctive behavioral phenotype. *Ment Retard Develop Dis Res Rev.* 2000; 6(2):142-147.

142. Shprintzen RJ. Genetics of pediatric heart disease. *Prog Ped Cardiol.* 2005;20(2):187-193.

143. Shprintzen RJ, Goldberg RB. Multiple anomaly syndromes and learning disabilities. In: Smith SD, ed. *Genetics and Learning Disabilities.* San Diego, Calif: College-Hill Press; 1986.

144. Waardenburg PJ. A new syndrome combining developmental anomalies of the eyelids, eyebrows and nose root with pigmentary defects of the iris and head hair and with congenital deafness. *Am J Hum Genet.* 1951;3:195.

145. Fraser GR. *The Causes of Profound Deafness in Childhood.* Baltimore, Md: Johns Hopkins University Press, 1976.

146. Bodurtha J, Nance WE. Genetics of hearing loss. In: Alberti PW, Ruben RJ, eds. *Otologic Medicine and Surgery.* New York, NY: Churchill Livingstone; 1988;831-853.

147. Tassabehji M, Newton VE, Read AP. Waardenburg syndrome type 2 caused by mutations in the human micro-ophthalmia (MITF) gene. *Nature Genet.* 1994;8:251-255.

148. Gorlin RJ, Toricello HV, Cohen MM. *Hereditary Hearing Loss and Its Syndromes.* New York, NY: Oxford University Press, 1995.

149. Konigsmark BW, Gorlin RJ. *Genetic and Metabolic Deafness.* Philadelphia, Pa: WB Saunders; 1976.

150. Cremers CWRJ, Hoagland GA, Kuypers W. Hearing loss in the cervico-oculo-acoustic (Wildervanck) syndrome. *Arch Oto-laryngol.* 1984;110:54–57.
151. Kirkham TH. Inheritance of Duane's syndrome. *Br J Ophthal-mol.* 1970;54:323.
152. Wettke-Schafer R, Kantner G. X-linked dominant inherited diseases with lethality in hemizygous males. *Hum Genet.* 1983;64:1–23.
153. Ruben RJ, Rapin I. Management of hearing-impaired and deaf infants and children. In: Alberti PW, Ruben RJ, eds. *Otologic Medicine and Surgery.* New York, NY: Churchill-Livingstone; 1988.

# Section 1.2

# *Exogenous Etiology*

## BACTERIAL AND VIRAL INFECTIONS

Among the known causes of hearing loss in newborns are infections that the mother suffers during pregnancy. Cyto-megalovirus (CMV) is the most common virus transmitted to a pregnant woman's fetus. Another is maternal rubella (MRub).

Postnatally, any infection causing high fevers may lead to a hearing loss; for example, measles, mumps, and scarlet fever. A significant cause during child and adult years is meningitis (Menin), both bacterial and viral. For some other infections, see Otitis Media and Lues in this Section.

### Frequency of Occurrence

CMV is estimated to account for one-third of congenital hearing losses, occurring in approximately 1 per 100 newborns, of whom about 10 to 15% develop hearing problems.[1]

Menin has been estimated in Western countries to cause from 3 to 10% of severe to profound sensorineural hearing loss in children.[2] The bacterial form is less frequent than the viral. However, since the introduction of the Meningitis C vaccine, in 1999, there has been a dramatic drop in new cases of Menin in those countries that apply it.[3]

The incidences of MRub and the childhood diseases occur sporadically, so their incidence rates vary too widely for any single rate to be representative.

## Etiology

Infections act to destroy CNS tissue. The nature and extent of the damage they cause depend on the specific organisms and the time in which they are active.

CMV is most likely to cause hearing losses when it occurs in the first 24 months.[4] MRub may negatively affect the fetus's hearing whenever it arises during pregnancy, although, like other infections, it probably is most deleterious to fetal auditory development in the first trimester.[5]

In childhood and adult infections, the nature and duration of an infection affect its consequences. Further factors influencing sequelae are the promptness and efficacy of medical treatment.

## Diagnosis

Hearing losses that develop as a result of congenital CMV sometimes go unrecognized. One reason is it tends to be asymptomatic and develops progressively after birth. Another reason is that the virus may cause mental retardation and cerebral palsy—conditions that are more likely to gain the attention of diagnosticians, especially if the hearing loss is a relatively mild one. A review of the literature recommends audiologic examination for infants showing any symptoms of CMV infection (e.g., purplish skin rash, jaundice, low birth weight, swollen lymph glands).[6]

## Management

With respect to the hearing loss, the usual management considerations apply. The other sequelae of infections require the attention of clinicians who are expert in their fields: audiologists and otologists for the hearing loss, educators for the learning disabilities, physicians for the medical conditions, speech-language pathologists for speech and language development, and so forth.[7]

With respect to MRub, preventive doses of gamma globulin given to pregnant women during rubella epidemics may avoid damage to the fetus. Similarly, vaccination against Menin has become available and, as with other measures taken during epidemics, it should be applied when conditions indicate.[8,9]

# MATERNAL BEHAVIOR DURING PREGNANCY

Maternal behavior during pregnancy may contribute to a neonate's hearing loss.

## Frequency of Occurrence

The numerous maternal behaviors that can affect a fetus's development create a moving target for any attempts to estimate incidence.

## Etiology

Ingestion of alcohol (fetal alcohol syndrome[10]), recreational drugs (cocaine, methamphetamine, and marijuana) and, possibly, nicotine and caffeine may affect the fetus's developing hearing ability.[11-13] Even the mother's noise exposure during pregnancy might affect the fetus's hearing ability.[14]

A pregnant woman's general health also poses a possible risk to her fetus. Medications taken during pregnancy can affect fetal auditory development. However, as the mother in such cases is taking prescribed medications, any hearing loss in her neonate could as well be attributed to the condition for which she is being medicated rather than to the medication. For example, antibiotics to combat gram-negative bacteria in the pregnant mother might contribute to hearing loss in the fetus that she is carrying.[15]

## Diagnosis

Neonatal screening will identify hearing losses but will not diagnose the cause(s). As recommended in other congenital hearing disorders, DNA analysis and thorough familial histories can be useful in assessing any genetic contributions. If these diagnostic procedures are negative, a searching review of maternal behavior during pregnancy may resolve doubts about the cause of a hearing loss.[16]

## Management

Prompt prescription of appropriate amplification can assist in avoiding the impact on speech and language development of a hearing loss.

## NOISE-INDUCED HEARING LOSS

Noise-induced hearing loss (NIHL) may be of any degree from mild to severe, depending, at least in part, on the length and extent of the noise exposure.[17]

## Frequency of Occurrence

Prolonged exposure to excessive noise levels probably represents the most frequent cause of new cases of hearing loss among working-age adults. More than 30 million Americans are exposed to hazardous sound levels on a regular basis in the workplace, in recreational settings, and at home.[18] The National Institute of Occupational Safety and Health recognizes NIHL as the second most frequently self-reported injury, and it recommends standards for safe noise-exposure in industry.[19]

## Etiology

NIHL damages hair cells in the cochlea and disrupts connections to higher auditory centers. Hair cells can recover within 48 hours, the usual duration of temporary threshold shift (TTS). Permanent threshold shift (PTS) occurs when noise levels overwhelm this self-repairing capability and when constant or cumulative exposures to noise levels exceed 75 to 80 dBA over long periods in susceptible ears.[20]

Current research finds different mechanisms lead to TTS than cause PTS. What is effective in preventing TTS appears to differ from what is effective in preventing PTS.[21]

Damage-risk criteria for NIHL include the noise's sound-pressure level, spectral characteristics, and duration of exposure. Other contributing factors affecting NIHL are individual susceptibility and exposure to solvents and heavy metals that may act synergistically or independently to affect hearing permanently.[22,23]

When played for extended periods at high volume, music playback instruments like the iPod and the Walkman pose risks to their users' hearing. Members of rock bands also face the same dangers. Those exposed to these conditions should be alert to symptoms of potentially hazardous effects: inability to hold a conversation with a person next to them while they are playing, misperceptions of consonants, and onset of prolonged tinnitus. These symptoms should warn users to reduce the playback volume, discontinue the devices' use, and/or avoid further exposure to loud sounds.[24]

## Diagnosis

Distinguishing acoustic trauma from the far more prevalent NIHL that occurs over time is essential. Acoustic trauma is more dramatic: its effect is an immediate hearing decrement after exposure to a noise of 120 dB SPL or more. Although hearing sensitivity sometimes returns in a period of hours or days, small amounts of permanent damage often remain and may increase susceptibility to future exposures. Organic changes resulting from chronic exposure to less intense noise levels are less definitive. There are signs of metabolic exhaustion—hair-cell deterioration and reduced energy carried by the cochlear fluids.[25]

Otoacoustic emissions (OAE) do not predict when a TTS becomes a PTS, but this procedure may have value in determining who is susceptible to NIHL. An individual's OAE following noise exposure might show early changes in outer hair cells, suggesting greater risk for NIHL. Conversely, however, a negative OAE does not mean that the individual is not susceptible to NIHL.[26]

## Management

Most NIHL can be prevented or limited with reasonable precautions. Limiting noise exposure can reduce the number of persons affected, and a vigorous hearing-conservation program can help to reduce NIHL.[27] The current standard with which employers in the United States must comply can be found in the final OSHA Hearing Conservation Amendment.[28]

Although federal agencies have set standards for industry to follow, some situations cannot be managed in that way. Military personnel in war zones and, occasionally, in training exercises may be exposed to sudden, extreme noise levels that cannot be anticipated and do not allow for preparations to prevent damage. Use of a high-frequency tone of moderate intensity just prior to the noise may activate the ear's defenses (i.e., stapedius muscle contraction) and prevent acoustic trauma.

### *Otoprotective Devices*

When excessive noise cannot be avoided, personal hearing-protective devices can attenuate the noise and reduce or eliminate its damage. Extremely high noise levels in industry (in excess of 120 dB SPL) may require a combination of engineering, administrative, and personal hearing-protective measures. The use of special earmuffs to protect against NIHL has been proposed, and the equipment is available.[29]

### *Medication*

Antioxidants that detoxify free radicals and agents that increase blood flow to the cochlea may protect or rescue hair cells, and drugs effective in animal studies may be effective in humans.[30]

The combination of magnesium and high doses of vitamins A, C, and E taken 1 hour before noise exposure and continued once daily for 5 days prevented PTS in guinea pigs. The combination seemed to avoid some inner-ear damage by blocking excessive free-radical activity when taken several days prior to noise exposure by Israeli soldiers.[31] Two recently tested medications—evadarone and revarsatrol—may prove to be effective in preventing damage or restoring functions, but results have been reported only in animals.[32]

At present, persons at risk should consult their health professionals about drugs and dietary supplements, follow a healthy lifestyle, and adopt a well-balanced diet.[33] Research holds out prospects for regeneration of hair cells. Although still in experimental phases, initial results appear promising.[34]

### *Monitoring*

Employees, military personnel, and others who have been exposed to intense noises should have their hearing tested at least annually. Such examinations can detect subtle changes in hearing sensitivity and alert clinicians to the need for steps to prevent further damage to hearing.[35,36]

# OTITIS MEDIA (OM) AND SEROUS OTITIS MEDIA (SOM)

OM refers to an acute infection of the middle ear. SOM, also referred to as middle-ear effusion, often results in a relatively common exogenous cause of childhood hearing loss.

## Frequency of Occurrence

During early childhood, 15 to 20% of children are estimated to experience recurrent OM; that is, three or more acute episodes in that period. The National Center for Health Statistics reports physician visits for OM rose from 10 million, in 1975, to over 25 million, in 1990.[37]

The incidence of OM in 125 consecutive infants admitted to the Infant Intensive Care Unit of a U.S. hospital was found to be 30%. Children under 2 years of age accounted for the highest rate of physician visits for OM. Surveys have found from 75 to 95% of all children have at least one episode of OM by 6 years of age.[38]

Although SOM does not lead inevitably to hearing losses, it causes them in a sizable portion of reported cases. Incidence rates, however, are strongly influenced by the treatment accorded. Prompt, effective resolution of the condition avoids hearing impairment.

## Etiology

OM is due to an infection and is characterized by fever, severe pain, and hyperemia. A mild hearing loss may be associated with it. If untreated, the acute form can lead to mastoiditis and facial-nerve involvement.[39]

SOM, by contrast, has few symptoms other than a fluctuating conductive hearing loss. It can persist for years without permanently damaging the middle ear, although hearing loss can occur fairly early after onset.[40]

Anything that interferes with the eustachian tube's opening may cause OM; for example, infection, allergy, blockage by enlarged adenoids, and congenital deformity. OM occurs most commonly in children largely because their eustachian tubes are smaller and shaped differently than adults (shorter and with relatively flaccid cartilage). Children with cleft palate are particularly susceptible to SOM because their palatal muscles that control the eustachian tube's opening are weaker.[41,42]

## Diagnosis

Among young children, early indicators of OM are signs that the children are experiencing pain, often by handling their ears in a vain attempt to curb the pain. Otoscopic examination confirms the existence of OM. Audiologic evaluation determines the extent to which the infection has impinged upon hearing.

EarCheck is a relatively inexpensive device for parents to determine if there is fluid in the middle ear. So far no studies of its usefulness have been published.[43]

## Management

If untreated or inappropriately managed, the fluid in the middle ear changes viscosity to a thickness that may resemble cement, at which point it earns the appellation "glue ear" also called adhesive OM—a condition difficult but possible to treat. It can cause a conductive hearing loss in the 60- to 70-dB range. When chronic, SOM can lead to cholesteatoma, which can result in a substantial hearing loss.

First, the infection or the allergy triggering the hearing loss must be treated, initially with antibiotics, antihistamines, and decongestants. Although SOM and acute OM do not lead inevitably to hearing loss, they may cause a 20- to 65-dB hearing loss before treatment. Prompt, effective resolution avoids long-term hearing impairment. One study reports that 80% of 108 children with SOM spontaneously recovered after 2 months.[44]

The Ear Popper—a nonsurgical device developed for home use—may also be useful in aspirating fluid accumulations. It delivers a constant, controlled stream of air into the nasal cavity, diverting air into the eustachian tube as the patient swallows. This ventilates the middle ear and, usually, eliminates conductive hearing losses promptly. It also treats barotrauma (injury due to atmospheric pressure).[45]

If these measures are unsuccessful or cholesteatoma has developed, surgical repair is usually next. Myringotomy attempts to relieve pressure, restore normal hearing, and prevent damage to the ossicular chain. A tube inserted in an incision in the eardrum provides ventilation and temporarily performs the function of the inadequately functioning eustachian tube. Adenoidectomy may also be needed, if enlargement of the adenoids interferes with the eustachian tube's equalizing middle-ear pressure.[46]

SOM patients with ventilation tubes may conduct normal activities, although they must keep water out of the ear canal with earplugs when showering, washing hair, and swimming. Because the ventilation tubes are not intended to be permanent, careful attention to how well they are tolerated and how soon the causes for them have been eliminated are essential.

After surgery, the hearing loss becomes the focus of treatment. A joint policy statement of American Academy of Family Physicians, American Academy of Otolaryngology-Head and Neck Surgery, and American Academy of Pediatrics Subcommittee on Otitis Media with Effusion urges cooperation between a pediatric otologist and a pediatric audiologist when a comprehensive audiologic examination reveals a conductive hearing loss.[47]

Middle-ear disease has been associated with speech and language delays. Early diagnosis and treatment can often prevent permanent hearing loss and its most severe consequences.[48] Efforts continue to develop a vaccine for OM. It could virtually wipe out childhood hearing loss from acute OM, greatly reducing the incidence of hearing loss in young children.[49]

## OTOTOXIC MEDICATIONS

Ototoxic medications are among the major *preventable* causes of hearing loss and contribute substantially to tinnitus.[50] As medications that entail risks of damaging hearing may be essential to maintaining health or even to preserving life, prudent and ethical practices do not ban their use but require care in their administration or choosing alternative therapies when feasible.[51]

### Frequency of Occurrence

Determining the extent of hearing loss resulting from ototoxic drugs faces several difficulties:

- There is no government-reporting requirement.
- Damage may not be manifest until well after a patient is discharged from the service providing the medication.

- Hearing losses may be confined to the higher frequencies and are only detected by audiometry. Damage to frequencies over 8000 Hz require special equipment not generally available to be detected.
- Relatively small losses, especially in children, can have significant consequences, although the aftereffects may be slow to appear.

The U.S. Department of Veterans Affairs estimates that over 100,000 veterans in 2002 received potentially ototoxic medications during their hospitalization.[52]

Hearing loss in children from platinum-based chemotherapy has long been underreported.[53] Researchers found 41 of 67 patients treated with platinum-based chemotherapy had a high-frequency hearing loss with onset beginning an average 135 days after chemotherapy. These delayed effects make it difficult to establish the relationship between drug administration and auditory-vestibular damage.[54] The National Cancer Institute's "Common Terminology Criteria for Adverse Events" (CTCAE) does not include high-frequency hearing loss, the range usually affected by chemotherapy, and its published accounts only report severe to profound losses.

## Etiology

The intake of chemicals other than as medication may be involved in causing hearing loss. Unlike the interest in potentially ototoxic medication, comparatively little research has been done on chemicals that may also be ototoxic. For example, long-term exposure to trichloroethylene (an industrial solvent) has been associated with hearing loss.[55]

Genetic factors appear to be determiners of which patients will sustain impairment from ototoxic medication—whether permanent or transient and to what degree depends on the medication. An existing hearing loss also increases the possibility that an ototoxic drug will lead to further damage, as will prior or concurrent ingestion of ototoxic medication.[56]

The potential for adverse auditory side effects increases when patients take more than one ototoxic drug or follow one with intense noise exposure; for example, some industrial products, like solvents, and some medications, like aminoglycosides, may combine to exacerbate hearing loss.[57] Similarly, aspirin's transient cochleotoxicity can produce permanent hearing loss when accompanied by prolonged exposure to high-intensity noise.

## Diagnosis

Tinnitus provides a warning sign of ototoxic hearing loss. Patients on a newly prescribed medication should be advised to report immediately the onset of tinnitus, although high-frequency tinnitus is not a reliable indicator of damage. Detecting incipient hearing loss due to ototoxic medications requires ongoing testing of hearing.[58]

Because the susceptible frequencies are at the high end, audiometry can be conducted in bedridden patients' rooms if ambient noise is primarily in the low frequencies. Long-term audiometry following a course of treatment with ototoxic drugs is essential to identify hearing loss of which the patient may be unaware and which may occur after termination of therapy.

Ultrahigh-frequency audiometry during and following treatment with ototoxic medication should be included in the examination, as some auditory changes occur in the 10- to 20-kHz range before affecting the lower frequencies.[59]

Observation protocols for vestibulotoxicity remain problematic. None are efficient, reliable or suitable for use with ill patients who are bedridden, and none are generally accepted.[60]

## Management

Ceasing the administration of an ototoxic or vestibulotoxic medication is the obvious first step in treatment, if doing so is feasible. Alternative therapies may be selected or the dosage may be reduced or pulsed.[61] Long-term audiometry following a course of ototoxic drug treatment should continue for at least one year after cessation of drug therapy, because many of the drugs that can damage hearing have a delayed effect. Audiometric monitoring and consistent follow-up will alert the clinician to necessary modifications in treatment regimens, if further hearing and vestibular signs of damage appear. Word-recognition testing should be periodically reassessed. Monitoring is critical to detect changes in hearing during treatment with ototoxic drugs.[62,63]

Aside from cessation or alteration of the drug regimen, the rehabilitation of patients suffering ototoxicity and vestibulo-toxicity does not differ from that provided for patients whose symptoms emanate from other causes. Counseling about avoiding further damage to the auditory and vestibular systems are as important in these as in other cases of auditory and vestibular damage. Patients should be advised that the damage might not be permanent, depending on the medication, the dosage, individual susceptibility, and the time over which it was administered.[64]

## PREMATURE BIRTH

Delivery before full term leaves the neonate underdeveloped and subject to many potential dangers.

### Frequency of Occurrence

The number of children born prematurely is estimated to be about 500,000 annually in the United States. Approximately 11% of Caucasian and Hispanic women and about 18% of non-White women have premature births.[65] What is not available are data on the proportion of hearing losses in such births.

### Etiology

Sensorineural hearing loss due to prematurity may result from the use of various ototoxic medications in fetuses with immature liver and renal functions. Other factors affecting the perinatal maternal environment, for example, infections, drugs, or trauma, account for a substantial portion of the cases for which a cause can be established.

Recommended incubator noise has been reduced to below 58 dBA.[66] However, ambient noise levels over 60 dBA have been reported.[67] Although acceptable levels for damage risk are met, infants in incubators are in poor health, often receiving ototoxic drugs, and remain exposed continuously for long periods; hence, they remain at risk of hearing loss.[68]

## Diagnosis

See Section 1, "Newborn Infant Screening."

## Management

Although the number of premature births may or may not have increased recently, what has increased is the ability to keep alive infants born prematurely and attention to potential risks of damage to their hearing. Such efforts will likely continue, reducing the potential for damaging infant hearing.

# PSEUDOHYPACUSIS (PSH)

PSH refers to emotionally based auditory problems. It is also called nonorganic, psychogenic, hysterical, or functional hearing loss. It may be labeled "malingering"—a pejorative term—when an individual deliberately falsifies the condition.[69]

## Frequency of Occurrence

Age, gender, or socioeconomic status does not appear to affect the prevalence of this condition, although malingering seems to be greater among males than females.[70] Prevalence rates are reported to be higher in military and veterans groups than in the general population.

## Etiology

The condition may reflect emotional problems or conscious attempts to gain some advantage.[71,72]

## Diagnosis

Patients cue a diagnosis of PSH when they (1) repeat half of spondee words correctly; (2) evince better hearing for speech than for pure tones; (3) give inconsistent responses to pure-tone audiometrics; and (4) fail to show a shadow curve in unilateral hearing loss when no masking is used.[73] Preferred testing for this condition does not require subjective responses; for example, auditory stapedial reflex, otoacoustic emissions, and auditory brainstem responses. Other tests include Lombard Voice Reflex, Stenger, Delayed Speech Feedback, and Bekesy audiometry.[74]

## Management

Once diagnosed, clinicians usually refer such patients to a mental-health facility or practitioner.

## SYPHILIS (LUES)

When Lues progresses into its latter stages, fluctuating hearing losses and vestibular disorders that mimic Meniere's disease arise.

## Frequency of Occurrence

In the United States in 2005, the U.S. Centers for Disease Control and Prevention estimated there were 8,724 cases—an increase over 2004 of almost 10%. The current rate in the U.S. general population is about 29 per million.[75]

## Etiology

Immediately postinfection, few symptoms appear. In the late stages of Lues, it attacks the CNS. Hearing losses and vestibular problems are among the significant consequences of CNS involvement.

## Diagnosis

Special blood tests clearly identify this disease.[76] Audiometric examinations may be difficult in patients who have advanced syphilis with its attendant CNS effects, which make the patient's cooperation difficult to obtain. Gait and balance disorders are usually apparent.

## Management

Regardless of the stage of its development, syphilis should be treated with medication to stabilize its effects. Once a CNS-attack stage has been reached, however, any resulting hearing and vestibular disorders that develop cannot be reversed.

# TRAUMATIC BRAIN INJURY

Traumatic brain injury (TBI) has grown as a problem, as medicine has become increasingly adept at keeping affected persons alive and as a result of battlefield injuries. Some portion of TBIs affects hearing ability and causes tinnitus.

## Frequency of Occurrence

It is estimated that nearly 2 to 5 million people in the United States suffer either a focal or diffuse head injury annually. The Afghanistan and Iraq conflicts have increased the prevalence of TBI countries involved in those conflicts, and with that increase in TBI prevalence is the likelihood of an increase in hearing impairments.

About half of soldiers recently admitted to a U.S. Veterans Affairs hospital for blast-related TBI had a sensorineural hearing loss and nearly two-thirds complained of tinnitus.[77] Similar prevalence data for the civilian population are not available.

## Etiology

The damage resulting from a TBI depends on the cerebral location and its extent.

## Diagnosis

Detection of brain damage is the province of the neurologist. However, the examination should include a thorough audiologic assessment.

## Treatment

When a hearing loss accompanies TBI, measures to counter its effects through amplification should be prescribed promptly. In addition to amplification, rehabilitation should include compensatory strategies.

Recent studies have roused the possibilities of limiting or reversing damage due to TBI, including the following:

- Progesterone given shortly after an injury appears to reduce the deleterious effects of trauma.[78]
- Research on regeneration of CNS tissue opens the possibilities that some of the devastating effects of TBI may be reversed (see Section 1.1).
- Treatment of persons who have entered vegetative and minimally conscious states have been reported to have recovered some functions by deep brain (thalamic) stimulation.[79]

Although not directly focused on hearing, these studies encourage the hope that, in time, hearing losses accompanying TBI may be alleviated or eliminated altogether.

# REFERENCES

1. Reports of infectious diseases are published periodically by the Centers for Disease Control. Access any year at http://www.cdc.gov/cmv/facts.htm

2. Kapur YP. Epidemiology of childhood hearing loss. In: Gerber SE, ed. *The Handbook of Pediatric Audiology*. Washington DC: Gallaudet University Press; 1996:3–14.

3. Meningitis and hearing loss. Retrieved September 2007 from http://www.deafnessresearch.org.uk

4. Fowler KB, Stagno S, Pass RF. Interval between birth and risk of congenital cytomegalovirus infection. *Clin Infect Dis*. 2004; 38:1035–1037.

5. Chess S, Korn SJ, Fernandez PB. *Psychiatric Disorders of Children with Congenital Rubella*. New York, NY: Brunner/ Mazel; 1971.

6. Schildroth, AN, Karchmer, MA. *Deaf Children in America*. San Diego, Calif: College-Hill Press; 1986.

7. American Academy of Pediatrics, *Redbook On Line*. Retrieved December 2006 from http://aapredbook.aappublications.org/cgi/content/extract/2006/1/3.113

8. Reisinger KS, Hoffman Brown ML, Xu J, et al. A combination measles, mumps, rubella, and varicella vaccine (ProQuad) given to 4- to 6-year-old healthy children vaccinated previously with M-M-RII and Varivax. *Pediatrics*. 2006;117:265–272.

9. Katz FA. Pediatrics. In: Gerber SE, ed. *The Handbook of Pediatric Audiology*. Washington DC: Gallaudet University Press, 1996:15–34.

10. Alpert JJ, Zuckerman BS. Prevention of fetal alcohol syndrome. *Pediatrics*. 1993;92(5):739.

11. French JH, Haddad RK, Rabe A, et al. Environmental toxins and mental retardation. In: Berg JM, ed. *Perspectives and Progress in Mental Retardation, Volume 11, Biomedical Aspects*. Toronto, Canada: International Association for the Scientific Study of Mental Deficiency; 1984.

12. Fried PA. Prenatal exposure to tobacco and marijuana: effects during pregnancy, infancy, and early childhood. *Clin Obstet Gynecol*. 1993;36:319–337.

13. Fried PA, Ferruci L. Cigarette exposure and hearing loss. *J Am Med Assoc*. 1998;280(11):963.

14. Etzel RA, Balk SJ, Bearer CF, et al. Noise: a hazard for the fetus and newborn. *Pediatrics*. 1997:100:724-727.
15. Ryback L, Matz GJ. Ototoxicity. In: Alberti PW, Rubin RJ, eds. *Otologic Medicine and Surgery*. New York, NY: Churchill Livingston; 1988.
16. Paul M, ed. *Occupational and Environmental Reproductive Hazards. A Guide for Clinicians*. Baltimore, Md: Williams & Wilkins; 1993.
17. Alberti, PW. Hearing conservation. In: Alberti PW, Ruben RJ, eds. *Otologic Medicine and Surgery*. New York, NY: Churchill Livingstone; 1988.
18. Noise-induced hearing loss. National Institute on Deafness and Other Communicative Disorders. Retrieved December 2004 from http://www.nidcd.gov
19. National Institute for Occupational Safety and Health. *Criteria for a Recommended Standard: Occupational Noise Exposure*. Public No. 98-126. Washington, DC: U.S. Department of Health and Human Services; 1998.
20. Schneider ME, Belyantseva IA, Azevedo RB, et al. Rapid renewal of auditory hair bundles. *Nature*. 2002;418(6900):837-838.
21. Nixon CW, Sommer HC, Cashin JL. Use of the aural reflex to measure ear protector attenuation in high level sound. *J Acoust Soc Am*. 1963 35(10): 1535-1543.
22. Cary R, Clarke S, Delie J. 1997. Effects of combined exposure to noise and toxic substances: critical review of the literature. *Ann Occ Hyg*. 41:455-465.
23. Fecther LD. Promotion of noise-induced hearing loss by chemical contaminants. *J Toxicol Environment Hlth*. 2003; 67(8-10):727-740.
24. Miller MH, Schein JD. What's all this noise? *Hear Loss*. 2006; 27(6):26-27.
25. Melnick W. Auditory effects of noise exposure. In: Miller MH, Silverman CA, eds. *Occupational Hearing Conservation*. New York, NY: Prentice-Hall; 1984.
26. Hochenburger E. A new objective, accurate and quick method to determine the damping effect of hearing protectors with the aid of the stapedial reflex. *XVIII International Congress of Audiology*, Prague: Czechoslovakia [Abstracts]; 1986:90.
27. Miller MH. Hearing conservation in industry. *Curr Opin Otol Head Neck Surg*. 1998;6:352-357.

28. Lipscomb DM, ed. *Hearing Conservation in Industry, Schools, and the Military*. San Diego, Calif: Singular; 1995.

29. Carter NL, French HT, LePage E, et al. Aural reflex eliciting ear-muffs for artillery gun crew. In: Carter N, Job RFS, eds. *Noise Effects '98. Proceedings of the 7th International Congress on Noise as a Public Health Problem*. Sydney, Australia: '98 Pty. Ltd; 1998.

30. Campbell KCM. Otoprotective agents sought for noise-induced hearing loss. *ASHA Leader*. 2004;3(5):16.

31. Leprell CG, Hughes; LF, Miller JM. Free radical scavenger vitamins A, C, and E plus magnesium reduce noise trauma. *Free Radical Bio Med*. 2007;42(9):1454–1463.

32. Tanaka K, Takemoto T, Sugahara K, et al. Post-exposure administration of edaravone attenuates noise-induced hearing loss. *Eur J Pharmacol*. 2005;522:116–121.

33. Seidman M, Babu S, Tang W, et al. Effects of resveratrol on acoustic trauma. *Otolaryngol Head Neck Surg*. 2003;129(5):463–470.

34. Salvi RJ, Chen L, Hasino E, et al. Regeneration of sensory and supporting cells: Relationship to physiological and psychophysical measures. In: Manley GA, Klump GM, Koppl C, et al. eds. *Advances in Hearing Research: Proceedings of the 10th International Symposium on Hearing*. Singapore: World Scientific Publishers, 1995.

35. Brookhouser PE. Prevention of noise-induced hearing loss. *Prev Med*. 1994;23:665–669.

36. Noise-induced hearing loss. Retrieved May 2000 from http://www.aafp.org/afp20000501/2749.html

37. Schapport SM. *Office Visits for Otitis Media: United States 1975–1990*. Report No. 214. Hyattsville, Md: National Center for Health Statistics; 1992.

38. Balkany TJ, Berman SA, Simmons MA, et al. Middle ear effusion in neonates. *Laryngoscope*. 1978;88:398–405.

39. Michaels L. Pathology of the external and middle ear. In: Alberti PW, Ruben RJ, eds. *Otologic Medicine and Surgery*. New York, NY: Churchill Livingstone; 1998.

40. Roark R, Berman S. Otitis media. In: Northern JL, ed. *Hearing Disorders*. Boston, Mass: Allyn & Bacon; 1996.

41. Castillo MP, Roland PS. Cleft palate. In: Roeser RJ, Valente M, Hosford-Dunn H, eds. *Audiology Diagnosis*. 2nd ed. New York, NY: Thieme; 2007.

42. Paradise JL, Bluestone CD. Early treatment of the universal otitis media of infants with cleft palate. *Pediatrics*. 1974;53:48-54.

43. EarCheck middle-ear monitor. Retrieved September 2007 from http://www.earcheck.com

44. Casselbrant ML, Brostoff LM, Cantekin EI, et al. Otitis media with effusion in pre-school children. *Laryngoscope*. 1985; suppl 95:428-436.

45. How can an EarPopper help you? Retrieved September 2007 from http://www.earpopper.com

46. Mattila PS, Joki-Erkkila VP, Kilpi T, et al. Prevention of otitis media by adenoidectomy in children younger than 2 years. *Arch Otolaryngol Head Neck Surg*. 2003;129:163-168.

47. American Academy of Pediatrics Subcommittee on Otitis Media with Effusion. Retrieved September 2007 from http://aap policy.aappublications.org/.

48. Rapin I. Conductive hearing loss effects on children's language and scholastic skills: a review of the literature. *Ann Otolaryngol Rhinol Laryngol*. 1979;88:3-12.

49. Cripps AW, Kyd J. Bacterial otitis media: current vaccine development strategies. *Immunol Cell Biol*. 2003;81:46-51.

50. Henley CM, Ryback LP. Ototoxicity in developing mammals. *Brain Res Rev*. 1995;20(1):10-16.

51. ASHA Guidelines. Audiologic management of individuals receiving cochleotoxic drug therapy. *Asha*. 1994;36(suppl 12):11-19.

52. Fausti SA, Wilmington DJ, Helt PV, et al. Hearing health and care: the need for improved hearing loss prevention and hearing conservation practices. *J Rehab Res Develop*. 2006;42(4):45-62.

53. Brummett RE. Drug-induced ototoxicity. *Drugs*. 1980;19:412-428.

54. Gratto MA, Salvi PV, Kamin BA, et al. Interaction of cisplatinum and noise on the peripheral auditory system. *Hear Res*. 1990;50:211-223.

55. Burg JR, Gist GI. Health effects of environmental contaminant exposure: an intrafile comparison of the trichloroethylene subregistry. *Arch Environmen Hlth*. 1999;54:231-241.

56. Hutchins TP, Cortopassi GA. Mitochondria and risk for deafness. *Am J Audiol*. 1995;4:12-14.

57. Brown JJ, Brummett RE, Meilhle MB, et al. Combined effects of noise and Kanamycin. *Arch Otolaryngol Head Neck Surg*. 1980;106:744-750.

58. Leigh-Paffenroth E, Reavis KM, Gordon JS, et al. Objective measures of ototoxicity. *ASHA Spec Interest Div 6, Perspect Hear Hear Disord: Res Diagnost.* 2005;9:10–16.

59. Fausti SA, Frey RH, Erickson DA, et al. A system for evaluating auditory function from 8000–20000 Hz. *J Acoust Soc Am.* 1979;66:1713–1718.

60. Dayal VS, Chait GE, Fenton SS. Gentamycin vestibulotoxicity. Long-term disability. *Ann Otol Rhinol Laryngol.* 1979;88: 36–39.

61. Fausti SA, Wilmington DJ, Helt PV, et al. Hearing health and care—the need for improved hearing loss prevention and hearing conservation practices. *J Rehab Res Develop.* 2005; 42:45–62.

62. Konrad-Martin D, Gordon JS, Reavis KM, et al. Audiological monitoring of patients receiving ototoxic drugs. *ASHA Spec Interest Div 6, Perspect Hear Hear Disord: Res Diagnost.* 2005;9:17–21.

63. Gordon JS, Phillips DS, Helt WJ, et al. The evaluation of insert earphones for high-frequency bedside ototoxicity monitoring. *J Rehab Res Develop.* 2005;42:353–362.

64. Konrad-Martin D, Wilmington DJ, Gordon JS, et al. Audiological management of patients receiving aminoglycoside antibiotics. *Volta Rev.* 2005;105(3):229–250.

65. Institute of Medicine, adviser to the nation to improve health. Retrieved September 2007 from http://www.iom.edu/

66. American Academy of Pediatrics Committee on Environmental Hazards. Noise pollution: neonatal aspects. *Pediatrics.* 1974;54:476.

67. Douek E, Dodson H, Banister L, et al. Effect of incubator noise on the cochlea of the newborn. *Lancet.* 1976;2:1110–1113.

68. Falk S, Farmer J. Incubator noise and possible deafness. *Arch Otolaryngol.* 1973;97:385.

69. Martin FN, Clark JG. *Introduction to Audiology.* 9th ed. Boston, Mass: Allyn & Bacon; 2006.

70. Burgoon DN, Buller DB, Woodall WG. *Nonverbal Communication: The Unspoken Dialogue.* New York, NY: Harper & Row; 1989.

71. Brooks DN, Goeghegan PM. Non-organic hearing loss in young persons: transient episode or indicator of deep-seated difficulty? *Br J Audiol.* 1992;26:347–350.

72. Johnson J, Weissman MM, Klerman GL. Service utilization and social morbidity associated with depressive symptoms in the community. *J Am Med Assn*. 1992;267:1478-1483.

73. Shoup AG, Roeser RJ. Audiologic evaluation of special populations In: Roeser RJ, Valente M, Hosford-Dunn H, eds. *Audiology Diagnosis*. 2nd ed. New York, NY: Thieme; 2007.

74. Martin FN. Pseudohypacusis. In: Katz J, ed. *Handbook of Clinical Audiology*. 5th ed. New York, NY: Lippincott Williams & Wilkins: 2002.

75. Syphilis Surveillance Report for 2005. Retrieved September 2007 from http://www.cdc.gov/std/Syphillis2005/default.htm

76. Northern JL, Downs MP. Medical aspects of hearing loss. In: Northern JL, Downs MP, eds. *Hearing in Children*. 5th ed. New York, NY: Lippincott Williams & Wilkins: 2002.

77. Lew H, Henry J. Auditory dysfunction in blast-related traumatic brain injury. *J Rehab Res Develop*. 2007;44(7):921-928.

78. Wright D, Kellermann A, Hertzberg V, et al. ProTECT: a randomized clinical trial of progesterone for acute traumatic brain injury. *Ann Emergen Med*. 2006;49(4):391-402.

79. Schiff N, Giacino J, Kalmar K, et al. Behavioural improvements with thalamic stimulation after severe traumatic brain injury. *Nature*. 2007;448:600-603.

# Section 1.3

# *Multiple Etiology*

## APLASIAS AND DYSPLASIAS

Aplasia refers to lack of development and dysplasia to abnormality of development. The two conditions occur in a number of syndromes that include hearing loss. In favor of conciseness, major examples of these anomalies are gathered in this Section. However, additional variations not specifically mentioned here probably exist.

In Alexander aplasia (AA), cochlear-duct differentiation at the level of the basal coil is limited, which affects development of the organ of Corti and the ganglion cells.

Alpert syndrome (APT) is characterized by abnormal facial appearance, spina bifida, and conductive hearing loss. The name alone may cause it to be confused with Alport syndrome (see Section 1.1) with which it shares no other features except hearing loss.[1]

Mondini dysplasia (MonD) is also called Mondini malformations. It is characterized by hearing disturbances and cataract, branchial cleft fistulae, and preauricular pits. It is closely related to several other syndromes; for example, Branchio-Oto-Renal and Kabuki (Niikawa-Kuroki), as well as with the others listed here.

Michel aplasia and dysplasia (MichelA/D) refer to the lack of differentiated inner-ear structures. In one form, it comprises the complete agenesis of the petrous portion of the temporal bone, with the auditory nerve and inner-ear structures absent.

In that case, the external and middle ear are unaffected. The condition is named for Pierre Michel.[2]

Scheibe aplasia (SA) involves agenesis of the inner ear. Its more descriptive name is Cochlear-saccular dysplasia or Pars Inferior dysplasia.

## Frequency of Occurrence

The aplasias and dysplasias are relatively rare conditions, each of them probably occurring in fewer than 1 in 10,000 live births. Estimating the incidences of these conditions is difficult, because similar malformations have been identified in other disorders, like Pendred, Waardenburg, Treacher-Collins, and Wildervaank syndromes, For that reason alone, more precise incidence rates for these conditions have dubious reliability unless the overlapping of symptoms are given careful account.

SA is thought to be the most common form of inner-ear aplasia.

## Etiology

The cause(s) of aplasias and dysplasias—aside from their being due to genetic defects—remain in doubt. The differentiation between aplasias and dysplasias probably depends on the time in development of the inner-ear structures when the mutation occurred.[3]

AA may be a phenotype rather than a genotype.
APT is assumed to be autosomal dominant.
MonD is thought to be congenital and probably X-linked.[4]

The vestibule and semicircular canals may develop normally, but perilymphatic fistulae commonly occur. The cochlea is deformed or missing, and the endolymphatic duct tends to be atypically large. These deformities may be unilateral or bilateral.

In MichelA/D, the defects are thought to result from an insult prior to the end of the third gestational week. Genetic studies of mouse models suggest that a number of different genes may cause these anomalies. Autosomal dominant inheritance has been hypothesized, but recessive inheritance is also regarded as likely in some cases.

SA is usually inherited as an autosomal recessive, nonsyndromic trait. Although the bony labyrinth and the superior portion of the membranous labyrinth are usually differentiated in patients with SA, the organ of Corti, the tectorial membrane, and Reissner's membrane tend to be deformed. Some infants with congenital rubella also display these deformities.

## Diagnosis

The hearing losses in these conditions may be unilateral. Audiologic testing followed by radiologic and MRI procedures usually confirm the inner-ear defects.

In MonD, the hearing loss is in the low to middle frequencies. Hearing at 8000 Hz and above usually remains intact. When ultrahigh-frequency hearing is not checked, MonD's characteristic audiometric configuration is often missed.

In MichelA/D, the hearing loss that accompanies this condition is usually moderate. Hearing loss is also a major component of Kabuki syndrome, in which it results in deafness due to the lack of sensorineural structures.

## Management

Audiologic testing is key for diagnosis of the aplasias and dysplasias, because counteracting the hearing loss is doable. Amplification with hearing aids and cochlear and brainstem implants should be considered.

For patients with AA who have a high-frequency hearing loss, their intact low-frequency hearing may justify use of conventional amplification or a hybrid cochlear implant.

Recognizing MonD can lead to treatment of a perilymphatic fistula that significantly helps prevent meningitis.

Conventional amplification and cochlear implants do not aid patients with MichelA/D, but vibrotactile devices, and implants directly into the auditory portion of the brains may provide assistance.

As in all aplasias and dysplasias, early application of treatment for a hearing loss has a high probability of avoiding speech and language delays.[5]

# AUDITORY PROCESSING DISORDER (APD)

APD refers to deficits in the perceptual processing of auditory stimuli and in the neurobiologic activity underlying these processes.[6] It may be further designated as (Central) Auditory Processing Disorder (CAPD).

## Frequency of Occurrence

When estimates of APD's incidence and prevalence are available, they will appear on the Web site of the National Institute of Deafness and Other Communicative Disorders.[7]

## Etiology

What causes APD is unknown. It may be due to a number of factors acting alone or in combination. In children, it has been associated with dyslexia, attention deficit disorder, autism spectrum disorder, specific language impairment, and pervasive developmental disorder or delay.[8]

## Diagnosis

A battery of behavioral and electrophysiologic tests have been developed.[9] A team approach to school-age children—audiologist, neuropsychologist, otologist, special educator, speech-language pathologist—should also involve the child's parents and teachers. In arriving at a diagnosis, the team will rule out other similarly appearing problems—especially attention deficit and hyperactivity disorders, which are often confused with APD.[10-12]

## Management

A variety of approaches may be tried to counteract the effects of APD. In classrooms, the teacher may wear a microphone that transmits her speech to the child wearing a headset, thereby reducing the effects of competing auditory stimuli. Adjusting room acoustics and the child's seating may also improve listening conditions.

Lessons that improve language skills and enhance auditory memory have been tried, and Auditory Integration Training (AIT) has also been offered. As yet, however, sufficient research does not support any of these techniques,[13] and AIT has provoked a technical report and a policy statement from the American Speech-Language-Hearing Association.[14,15]

## AUDITORY NEUROPATHY (AN)

AN is a recently adopted term also called Auditory Dyssynchrony. Either term refers to normal otoacoustic emissions, absent or abnormal auditory brainstem responses, absent acoustic reflexes, and poor speech discrimination.[16]

## Frequency of Occurrence

AN is a relatively rare condition, estimated to occur at a rate of about 1 or fewer per 10,000 population.[17] However, the relatively new awareness of this condition suggests cases will be identified at an increased rate.[18]

## Etiology

AN results from a combination of disturbances of the CNS from the axon terminal of the inner hair cells to the auditory brainstem.[19]

The hearing loss tends to be mild at first and slowly progressive to severe and even profound levels.[20]

## Diagnosis

An absent or abnormal auditory-brainstem response and normally functioning outer hair cells suggests a diagnosis of AN. Additionally, middle-ear muscle response is characteristically absent, and word recognition in quiet is out of proportion to pure-tone sensitivity. The diagnosis is further bolstered by absence of auditory-nerve action potential and may be confirmed by MRI.[21]

## Management

First attention must be given to dealing with the cause(s). The clinician can then consider management of the residual hearing capacity.

For children with AN, conventional hearing aids give mixed results. Some success has been reported with devices that improve the signal-to-noise ratio, like FM systems. Cochlear implants also give mixed, though generally favorable, results.[22,23]

## AUTOIMMUNE INNER-EAR DISEASE

Autoimmune inner-ear disease (AIED) arises from inflammation of the inner ear caused by the body's immune system attacking cells in the inner ear. It is a relatively new clinical entity, first identified in 1979.[24]

## Frequency of Occurrence

The National Institute of Allergy and Infectious Diseases (NIAID) estimates AIED accounts for less than 1% of all cases of hearing loss and vertigo.[25] However, prevalence estimates for this condition may be sizable underestimates, as some cases of bilateral Meniere's disease—which NIAD categorizes as one of the autoimmune diseases—and some portion, at least, of idiopathic sudden sensorineural hearing losses and possibly some other conditions should be included.

## Etiology

AIED is a fluctuating cochlear disorder whose potential for auditory recovery is unpredictable.[26] Contrary to the belief that the inner ear cannot be attacked by its own immune system, it now appears that the perisacular tissue surrounding the endolymphatic sac can provoke an autoimmune reaction as if attacked by a virus. There may also be causal factors as yet unidentified.

AIED is a poorly understood syndrome. Persons with this condition present with sudden, idiopathic, rapidly progressive sensorineural hearing losses that may be unilateral or bilateral. They may fluctuate over a period of weeks or months, and vestibular symptoms are present in approximately half of the patients.

Research on the etiology of this condition is hampered by its low incidence, its episodic nature, failures to recognize it, and the recentness of its discovery. Furthermore, persons with AIED may have more than one type of autoimmune disease or genetic defect. As noted above, some percentage of patients diagnosed with Meniere's disease, especially those with bilateral symptoms, may instead have AIED. The diagnosis is important to treatment, as patients with AIED tend to respond well to corticosteroid therapy.

## Diagnosis

Diagnoses are based on the patient's history, physical examination, audiologic and vestibular examinations, and blood tests. Western Blot Immunoassay for Heat Shock Protein-70 antibodies identifies rapidly progressive sensorineural hearing loss in a sizable number of cases.[27]

## Management

When diagnosis is doubtful, a medical regimen for AIED is recommended because the condition may be reversible and spontaneous recovery is possible.[16] It is usually treated initially with a variety of medications, among which steroids constitute the most favored medical response that gives relief to some patients with AIED. If the response to steroids is favorable, a cytotoxic chemotherapy, like cytoxan or methotrexate, may be used on a long-term basis.[28,29]

Some patients (e.g., diabetics) cannot be treated with steroids. Hyperbaric oxygen therapy is then an option, though results appear inconsistent.[30,31]

For patients who do not respond to drug and other medical therapy and whose hearing loss persists, amplification is recommended. Fully digital hearing aids should be considered because they can be reprogrammed as the patient's hearing loss changes.

If the hearing loss becomes profound, a cochlear implant may be prescribed. However, AIED's fluctuating nature requires that clinicians take a conservative approach to recommending cochlear implants, as the potential exists for recovery from or lessening of the hearing loss. If clinicians prescribe cochlear implants, they should advise patients with the possibility that the device will prevent the return of normal hearing.[32] The National Institute on Deafness and Other Communicative Disorders and the American Academy of Otolaryngology-Head and Neck Surgery Foundation cosponsor a multicenter clinical trial named Otolaryngology Clinical Trial Cooperative Group to uncover the cause of AIED and to evaluate drug therapies. As with the study of its etiology, the rarity of AIED makes research on its treatment difficult but worthwhile, as it may lead to better understanding of other sensorineural hearing losses.

## BRANCHIO-OTO-RENAL SYNDROME (BOR)

BOR is distinguished by branchial clefts, fistulas, cysts, and malformation of the pinnae and preauricular pits of the sinuses. Hearing impairments and kidney dysfunctions are common.

## Frequency of Occurrence

BOR probably occurs in about 1 per 40,000 live births.

## Etiology

The heritability of this congenital syndrome remains undetermined. It probably is caused by mutations within a genomic interval of 156 kB.

## Diagnosis

Three-fourths of BOR patients are estimated to have a hearing loss: about a third are conductive, a fifth are sensorineural, and the remainder mixed.

## Management

Providing appropriate amplification for the hearing loss early is the most rewarding measure in the rehabilitation of this condition. As with all syndromes, attention should be directed to the accompanying disabilities, especially renal failures that can be life-threatening. Genetic counseling should be made available to affected persons and their families.

# CHARGE ASSOCIATION

CHARGE Association (CA) is a syndrome whose acronym indicates its characteristics: *C*oloboma, *H*eart defects, *A*tresia of the choanae, *R*etarded growth, *G*enital hypoplasia, and *E*ar anomalies.

## Frequency of Occurrence

CA is estimated to occur in 1 in 12,000 live births.[33] Mild to profound sensorineural hearing losses occur in about 8 of 10 CA cases.[34] When 4 of the 6 characteristics appear together, diagnosis is confirmed.

## Etiology

The initials of the syndrome indicate the conditions involved in this syndrome. The ear anomalies may include hypoplasia of the external ear, hearing loss, a Mondini-type deformity, and absence of semicircular canals.[35] In addition to these symptoms, CA patients may have vestibular dysfunctions.[36]

CA occurs in both genders, all races, and all socioeconomic groups. The nature of inheritance—if it is inherited rather than arising from damage in utero—has not been established. The tiny incidence of the condition makes aggregating sufficient cases for genetic research difficult, amplifying the problems in determining its cause.[37]

## Diagnosis

The mix of disabilities in CA complicates audiologic evaluation. With four or more of the symptoms present at birth, the diagnosis of CA is usually made. Among other conditions with which CA may be confused is Usher syndrome (deafblindness).

## Management

Some of CA's structural anomalies may be amenable to surgical correction. Other aspects require medical care to maintain the patient's viability and to prevent deterioration of affected functions.[38]

In all cases, providing early amplification for the expected hearing loss is a critical step. It should be undertaken as early as feasible.[39]

# CONNEXIN 26 AND 30

Different mutations in the same gene can be associated with both dominant and recessive hearing loss. Connexins are membrane proteins that are primarily involved in intercellular communication. Connexin 26 (Cx26) and 30 (Cx30) cause the most common genetic forms of nonsyndromic hearing loss.[40]

## Frequency of Occurrence

The Cx26 and Cx30 mutations are heterozygous, and they are associated with several syndromes—for example, Keratitis-Ichthyosis-Deafness syndrome—which means that a single incidence-rate estimate for Cx-26 and Cx-30 defects would be misleading. They are involved in a number of syndromes.[41] Also, different national rates for their incidence have been reported for mutations in the GJB2 gene, which contains instructions for Cx26—mutations occurring most frequently in Caucasians, Ashkenazic Jews, and some Asian groups.[42-44]

## Etiology

Cx26 and Cx30 work together to form the cochlea's gap junctions and facilitate intercellular communication.[45] When they function properly, they encode gap-junction channels that connect adjacent cells and allow passage of cytoplasmic ions and small molecules.[46,47] More than 20 connexin subtypes have been identified in humans. Some connexin mutations induce hearing loss and may be responsible for a large amount of nonsyndromic congenital hearing loss in children.[48]

Nonsyndromic cases with hearing loss are not free of other disorders. But as other disorders are not due to the gene causing the hearing loss, they do not appear to be a part of a syndrome. Thirty-eight loci for dominant, nonsyndromic deafness have been mapped and 11 genes have been identified.

The recessive nature of these connexin disorders—when they are recessive—impairs permeability of cochlear structures.[49] Exogenous factors influence some cases.[50]

## Diagnosis

Genetic testing provides the basis for distinguishing aspects of this syndrome.[51]

## Management

As more molecular mechanisms are discovered for the effects of deafness-linked Cx26 mutations, the distinctions may assist clinicians to tailor therapeutic strategies to achieve best outcomes.

When Cx30 is missing, research with mice suggests that hair-cell depletion may be overcome and hearing restored by adding extra Cx26. Supplying a drug to boost production of Cx26 protein might provide similar results in the human instance. Although the majority of these genetic mutations cause recessive hearing loss, a few have been found to be dominant, in which case the hearing loss may be of any degree, ranging from moderate to profound. Such phenomena illustrate the nascent state of genetic research.

Research suggests a rationale for future therapeutic strategies to rescue cell death by G45E mutation by altering the $[Ca^{2+}]$ and/or binding affinity within the cochlea. Identifying more molecular mechanisms for the effects of deafness-linked Cx26 mutations may assist therapeutic strategies that achieve maximum clinical outcomes based on Cx26 mutations.[52]

# DOWN SYNDROME AND THE TRISOMY ABERRATIONS

Down syndrome (DS) is marked by developmental delays, characteristic features of the face, head, neck, and hands, and a mild congenital hearing loss.[53]

DS is named for J. L. H. Down, the physician who first described it.[54] DS is also known as Trisomy 21, the best known of the chromosome disorders. Trisomy 13 (Edwards' syndrome) and Trisomy 18 (Patau syndrome) are two related, but much less frequent variants of DS.

## Frequency of Occurrence

Estimates of the overall incidence of DS hover around 1 per 800 live births. This rate is affected by the age of the mother at conception: before 35 years of maternal age, the estimated incidence rate is about 1 per 1,000; from 35 to 40 years it rises to about 1 per 385; from 40 to 45 years, it reaches 1 per 106; and from 45 years of age and older it balloons to 1 per 30 live births.

The most common form of DS—about 90 to 95%—is Trisomy 21. The remaining 5 to 10% divide between the chromosomal anomalies Mosaicism and translocation.

The incidence of Patau is estimated to be about 1 per 7,600 and Edwards' to be slightly higher at an estimated 1 per 7,500 live births.[55]

## Etiology

DS results from extra genetic material. Instead of inheriting 23 chromosomes pairs from each parent, the neonate with DS has an extra chromosome (the "tri" in trisomy), which affects cell division and CNS development in utero.[56]

The hearing loss is frequently conductive and is associated with anomalies of the external ear and atresia of the auditory canals. Intellectual slowing commonly occurs.

## Diagnosis

Diagnosis of DS can be made in utero by ultrasound. DS is readily identified in newborns by noting its prominent physical characteristics.[57]

A variety of malformations of the ossicular chain, outer ear, middle ear, and nasopharynx, often with concomitant conductive hearing loss, characterize patients with DS.[58] They tend to have pinnae that are smaller and lower set than usual.[59] Ear canals are often stenotic, and malformations of the middle-ear structures have been reported.[60] DS also features excessive cerumen.[61]

Inner-ear malformations that involve both the cochlear and the vestibular portions do occur, but are infrequent.[62] However, when early onset sensorineural hearing loss similar to presbycusis occurs, it is considered significant and illustrative of DS. Its occurrence suggests that patients with DS exhibit accelerated aging, not only of the auditory systems, but also of the visual system and cognitive functions as well.[63,64]

## Management

Periodic monitoring is essential to patients with DS to detect and treat ear infections and to adjust any treatment for hearing losses they may have. Their tendency to conductive hearing losses is due to the narrowed eustachian tube and ear anomalies that characterize babies with DS and make them unusually susceptible to otitis media and serous otitis media. To avoid acquired hearing losses, management steps are the same as those for otitis media (see Section 1.2).[65,66]

The March of Dimes maintains a list of support groups on its Web site.[67]

# IDIOPATHIC SUDDEN SENSORINEURAL HEARING LOSS

Idiopathic, sudden sensorineural hearing loss (ISSNHL) ranks high among the difficult clinical conundrums. Patients with ISSNHL usually present with demands for relief, and much of the literature urges prompt treatment.

## Frequency of Occurrence

The incidence of ISSNHL is about 1 per 5,000 annually. Studies suggest that between 5 and 25 per 100,000 persons in the United States will suffer ISSNHL in any year.[68]

ISSNHL is predominantly unilateral. In about 7 in 10 cases, it is accompanied by tinnitus. An estimated 5 in 10 patients also suffer vertiginous attacks.[69]

Its incidence is far greater in adults than among children, with average age at onset between 40 to 50 years, and the majority of ISSNHL cases occurring in persons over 40 years old.[70]

Although the estimated incidence rates are relatively small, the number with ISSNHL amounts to about 65,000 persons annually in the United States. These estimates are for *reported cases*, which probably underestimate the actual rate, because many people do not seek medical assistance when the hearing loss is mild and their cases may not be brought to the attention of professionals when hearing recovers spontaneously after an attack.

## Etiology

The cause or causes of ISSNHL usually remain idiopathic despite assiduous efforts to identify etiology. Conductive losses from sharp changes in atmospheric pressure (aerotitis media), buildup of obstructive cerumen, ossicular-chain disruption, and swimmer's ear—all of which are usually self-limited, easily repaired, quickly reversed, and readily identified; thus, they are neither idiopathic nor sensorineural.

Exposure to a brief loud noise can cause a temporary threshold shift that is sensorineural (see NIHL in Section 1.2). Like conductive losses, such hearing losses are usually temporary, but with further noise exposure may result in permanent sensorineural hearing loss that a reasonably careful history correctly diagnoses. Nonetheless, their etiology can often be readily identified, so they are not idiopathic.

## Diagnosis

When a loss is sudden and sensorineural, its causation may be difficult or impossible to establish definitively, hence the *idiopathic* in ISSNHL. The published research emphasizes the difficulties in establishing an accurate diagnosis and prognosis for sudden hearing loss in about one of three cases.[71]

In addition to thorough audiologic and otologic examinations, other aspects of the patients' health should be examined and potential sources of hearing loss investigated; for example, brain scans and blood analyses. If these tests uncover a cause, the ISSNHL no longer is idiopathic, so treatment indicated by the new diagnosis shifts to management of that cause.

When the patient's hearing measures 70 dB HL or better, the remission possibilities are high.[72] Similarly rising and mid-frequency audiometric curves predict spontaneous recovery more frequently than sloping or flat configurations.[73]

Although most cases of ISSNHL are unilateral, bilateral cases have been reported.[74,75] When sudden deafness is bilateral, specific causes often have been diagnosed, typically instances of systemic disease.[76] A retrospective analysis of 324 cases found 16 patients (4.9%) with bilateral losses, of whom 6 were diagnosed with diabetes mellitus, 7 with hypertension or cardiovascular disease, and 3 remained idiopathic.[77]

## Management

Spontaneous recovery complicates rehabilitation planning in the interval between onset of the condition and beginning remediation. To be accepted as salutary, treatment must succeed better than the rates for spontaneous recovery, which occur in about one-third of cases. The proportion of cases enjoying spontaneous recovery declines after 30 days, with little hope for regaining hearing spontaneously after 6 months.[78]

Results of an 8-year prospective study of 225 patients concluded that the longer treatment is delayed, the poorer the recovery.[79] However, to date, no single treatment for ISSNHL has achieved success greater than that for spontaneous recovery.

### *Medical and Surgical Treatment*

In a study of short-term oral steroid treatment, hearing in the treated group improved by 29 dB HL compared to 11 dB HL for untreated cases. However, the expected rate of spontaneous recovery was unchanged.[80]

Magnesium added to steroids, but not antiviral drugs, were found to increase the rate of recovery somewhat.[81] A double-blind study that added vitamin E to the magnesium, steroid, and carbogen-inhalation therapy reported the combination significantly improved hearing for a majority of the patients.[82] Despite success of steroid therapies, alone or in combinations with other chemicals, questions about their use remain.[83]

## *Amplification*

Once medical or surgical treatments are deemed inappropriate, the patient should be offered amplification and auditory training. When the normal or better-hearing ear of an individual with unilateral loss is exposed to environmental noise, the ability to communicate is seriously reduced; in effect, under such conditions, the person is functioning with a significant bilateral hearing loss.

The time to amplify may depend on patient resistance and economics. The odds favoring spontaneous recovery justify a delay of 60 to 90 days, but a longer wait would be inadvisable in view of the handicap imposed and its isolating effects on social and occupational interactions.

Patients may resist suggestions to try a hearing aid, if it means to them they will not recover their hearing. Most patients will accept a hearing aid when told that its gain can be adjusted as hearing improves and its use discontinued if hearing returns to normal.

The style of hearing aid selected for patients must be consistent with their ability to manage the components easily and comfortably. Very small, completely in-the-canal instruments that use tiny batteries may not be appropriate for elderly persons with limited dexterity and poor vision. For them, a full-shell in-the-ear or an open-mold behind-the-ear hearing aid may be preferred.

Should the affected ear receive the aid? Or should the choice be among contralateral-routing-of-offside-signals aid (CROS), bone-anchored hearing aid (BAHA), and FM systems?[84] The indications and limitations of each system should be presented to the patient. If the affected ear has usable residual hearing, the audiologist should consider a hearing aid for that ear. If the affected ear has a profound hearing loss and word-recognition scores poorer than 20%, a CROS, transcranial CROS, or BAHA may offer a better solution.

In a CROS fitting, a microphone on the side of the affected ear electronically routes sounds originating on that side to an amplifier and receiver mounted near the normal or better-hearing ear, thus directing the sounds into the normal or better-hearing ear by tubing or a nonoccluding earmold that extends into the open ear canal. The object is to pick up sounds on the side of the affected ear and route them to the good ear, thus overcoming the head-shadow effect.

Some patients have reported mixed satisfaction with CROS amplification, although the majority of responses have been negative. The originator of the transcranial version reported a success rate of 25% in patients with severe to profound unilateral hearing loss.[85]

Personal FM systems that provide an improved signal-to-noise ratio in difficult listening environments are alternatives or additions to CROS aids. The transcranial CROS may be another option for persons with ISSNHL who have sustained severe-to-profound unilateral losses but have excellent hearing in the better-hearing ear. If the better-hearing ear has only a mild high-frequency hearing loss, conventional CROS aids may be recommended.[86]

The U.S. Food and Drug Administration has approved the BAHA for persons with single-sided deafness. BAHA is a cochlear stimulator that transmits auditory stimuli via bone conduction to the contralateral cochlea. This requires the surgical implantation of a 4-mm titanium fixture behind the affected ear. A multi-institutional study has shown greater patient satisfaction and improved communication with a BAHA than with a CROS.[87]

## Counseling

ISSNHL patients need counseling. They should have full explanations of the condition, its potential for spontaneous recovery and, if the loss persists, the treatment options.

The clinician should discuss fully and empathetically patients' desires to recover lost hearing. If told by one expert that hearing cannot be restored, many patients will shop for other more optimistic opinions. That is why clinicians should advise patients that, once the permanence of the hearing loss becomes likely, rehabilitation becomes an option and should counter any fears that rehabilitation may prevent later recovery of hearing.[88]

## *Monitoring*

Periodic audiologic examinations should not be overlooked. Partial recovery can occur in small steps that might be missed by patients. Further changes in hearing, both in the originally affected and the contralateral ear, can be useful in determining treatments formerly ignored and to identify possible causes originally rejected. For those reasons, serial pure tone audiometry and word-recognition testing appear wise.

## KERATITIS-ICHTHYOSIS-DEAFNESS SYNDROME (KID)

KID comprises ocular defects, including progressive blindness due to inflammation of the cornea (keratitis), and congenital hearing loss. Various other manifestations have been reported in association with KID, depending on the type of inheritance and degree of penetrance.

## Frequency of Occurrence

KID is a rare condition. No significant gender, racial, or ethnic influences have been reported.

## Etiology

KID appears to cover two modes of inheritance—one autosomal dominant and the other recessive—and one in which the genetic mutation leading to this cluster of conditions appears to be spontaneous, as other similarly affected relatives are not found in several of the reported cases.

## Diagnosis

The dominant characteristics, keratitis and deafness, present no difficulty in diagnosing. There are additional ectodermal defects in most cases—like dry, scaly skin—defects that are evident.

## Management

The hearing loss requires prompt attention, relying on amplification and other strategies to overcome potential impediments to speech, language, and social development.

# MENIERE'S DISEASE

Meniere's disease (MenDis) consists of a combination of hearing loss, vertigo, and tinnitus. It may also be accompanied by a sensation of fullness in the affected ear. It is named for the physician who first recognized it in 1861.

## Frequency of Occurrence

The prevalence of MenDis has been estimated to be the third most common inner-ear disorder after presbycusis and noise-induced hearing loss. Its occurrence has been variously estimated to be between 50 and 218 per 100,000.[89-91]

In about 70 to 80%, the hearing loss initially occurs unilaterally. Involvement of the unaffected ear—reaching about 40% after 15 years—often occurs as the disease progresses.[92] A higher prevalence of MenDis occurs in populations screened for migraine.[93]

## Etiology

MenDis has been attributed to many etiologies—food allergies, endocrine insufficiencies, vascular disease, syphilis, viral infection, and genetic factors—but none has gained consensus. It is now considered a disease of the membranous inner ear, attributable either to excessive endolymphatic fluid, causing Reissner's membrane to become distended, or to an injury of the fluid-absorption system. It has been postulated that Reissner's membrane may perforate during the acute attack and reattach itself between attacks.[94]

Because of the excess production or poor absorption of fluid, MenDis is often called endolymphatic hydrops, the assumed histopathologic hallmark of MenDis. However, Danish scientists have made an intriguing discovery (as yet unconfirmed) that the endolymphatic sac produces saccia, a hormone that plays a role in regulating the sodium level in the bloodstream.[95] This finding has led to the possibility of blocking the hormone's release with medication.[96]

## Diagnosis

The characteristic audiometric configuration in the early stages of MenDis is a rising curve. As the frequency increases, the hearing loss decreases. This contour has also been called a "reverse slope," as high-frequency hearing losses are by far the more frequent among persons suffering hearing loss. A much lower than expected word-recognition score often accompanies the pure-tone loss. High-frequency sensitivity tends to be normal in the early stages, but more lower and middle frequencies are involved as the disease progresses, leaving the patient with a "flat" or sloping audiometric configuration.

In MedDis, the hearing loss may vary from mild to severe. As MenDis progresses, the hearing loss usually becomes severe, ranging from 70 to 90 dB, and is accompanied by a roaring tinnitus with pronounced low-frequency components. These symptoms occur paroxysmally, with their duration varying from 20 minutes to several hours or days. Patients with MenDis usually have a premonition of vertigo that enables them to cease dangerous activities (such as driving) before its onset.

A complete audiologic evaluation of the patient suspected of having MenDis should include electrocochleography and electronystagmography.[97] A glycerol test is believed to aid diagnosis, but patients find it uncomfortable so it has largely been abandoned. The electrical responses of the cochlea and the assessment of vestibular function, with both positional and caloric stimulation, also provide important information for diagnosis and monitoring of treatment.[98]

In the early stages, MenDis usually presents as a unilateral, primarily low-frequency sensorineural hearing loss. However, lesions of the auditory nerve must be ruled out. Auditory brainstem responses and MRIs with contrast are necessary to rule out space-occupying lesions before the diagnosis of MenDis is established.

Differential diagnosis requires ruling out migraine-associated dizziness, as there is a higher prevalence of MenDis in a population screened for migraine than in the general population and vice versa.[99-101] The overlapping symptoms—vertigo or dizziness, tinnitus, and hearing loss—suggest an underlying link between the two pathologies.[102]

Audiologic and vestibular tests—such as electrocochleography and rotational-chair stimulation—provide limited diagnostic assistance.[103] Serial audiometry over time, along with vestibular findings and the case history combine to provide the strongest basis for a differential diagnosis.[104] Abnormal vestibular symptoms help to reinforce the differential diagnosis, but a clear pattern of progressive hearing loss is the principal criterion for differential diagnosis.[105]

The possibility that both conditions coexist further complicates diagnosis, especially in their prodromal stages. The expanded treatment options that arise from the differentiation, which include vestibular and balance rehabilitation, improve greatly the management outcomes.

## Management

The management of MenDis remains problematic. Initial treatment is conservative and a variety of medications provide symptomatic relief, but its severity usually prompts an immediate response. However, no single medical or surgical treatment has gained wide acceptance.[106]

A program of vestibular and balance rehabilitation training can have positive results for both MenDis and migraine-associated dizziness. The program is most useful in patients with MenDis following aggressive, destructive surgical or chemical procedures.[107]

This MenDis's paroxysmal character creates a conundrum for research and treatment. Emotional and/or physical stresses are known to trigger individual attacks of vertigo, hearing loss, and tinnitus. During acute attacks, patients' markedly reduced ability to discriminate speech and the accompanying vertigo challenge efforts to prescribe amplification and direct hearing rehabilitation.[108]

Between attacks in the early stages, auditory function may be normal or near-normal, but the fear of another attack often leaves the patient psychologically compromised. Further complicating management, the hearing loss is accompanied by loudness recruitment, narrowed range of comfortable loudness, and severe acoustic distortions. Digital amplification provides needed flexibility to counter hearing fluctuations.

Surgery may be undertaken for patients whose vertiginous attacks become disabling; these include the endolymphatic shunt.[109] A study compared this procedure to a sham operation and concluded that the 70% improvement in both treated and control groups was probably due to a placebo effect.[110] In extreme cases, severing the vestibular portion of the eighth nerve might be an option, if no usable hearing remains.[111]

Chemical ablation of hair cells in the vestibular labyrinth with intratympanic injections of gentamycin is another approach that claims success with low side effects.[112,113]

The Meniett device, a portable low-intensity alternating pressure generator, has been tried to alleviate the symptoms of MenDis.[114] In a study of 67 patients with unilateral MenDis assigned randomly to treatment or a control group, treatment was effective for at least 4 months in controlling severity and number of vertigo attacks.[115]

# OTOSCLEROSIS

Otosclerosis (OTO)—also known as otospongiosis—is a common cause of gradual hearing loss in adults, first identified by Politzer, in 1893.[116] It is progressive, with an unpredictable course.

## Frequency of Occurrence

OTO is one of the commonest causes of hearing loss in adults. Its frequency varies by age, race, and sex.[117] Clinical OTO increases with age, affects Caucasians more than other racial groups, and develops in women more than men.

## Etiology

The cause of OTO remains obscure, though family histories suggest an autosomal dominant transmission. Furthermore, there may be several genetic types. Exogenous causes of OTO, like measles virus infection, have also been suggested.[118]

Two types of OTO have been identified: histologic and clinical. The former has no apparent symptoms, being diagnosed by sectioning of the temporal bones. Hearing loss marks the clinical type, which is usually conductive, affecting the ossicles, and less frequently is sensorineural.[119]

OTO is bilateral in about 9 of 10 females and about 8 of 10 males. Clinical onset during pregnancy has been reported to be between 10 to 17% of females with OTO. It becomes more clinically apparent in females after pregnancy, which seems to accelerate its progression.[120] The hearing loss may worsen during periods of hormonal-endocrine changes, which may explain, at least in part, the discrepancy in gender incidence.[121]

In most cases, the onsets of hearing loss and tinnitus occur between 15 and 45 years. As it progresses, sensory involvement may be secondary to the footplate lesion or to a primary otosclerotic lesion in the cochlea. The latter may result from toxic metabolites released during the otosclerotic process, reduced blood supply to the lateral wall of the cochlea, or extension of the otosclerotic lesion to the cochlear duct, causing disruption of electrolyte composition and alteration of the basilar membrane biomechanics.[122]

Tinnitus is present in a majority of otosclerotic patients— the reported occurrence of which varies between half to over three-quarters of those with the clinical form. When the inner ear is involved, bouts of dizziness and imbalance may also occur.[123]

## Diagnosis

The onset of OTO is subtle and insidious. Because the hearing loss develops slowly, patients are often unaware of its initial onset. They may experience tinnitus long before they recognize a lessened hearing ability. The air-bone gap arouses suspicion of OTO, especially in patients emerging from their teens. At first, the loss occurs more in the lower frequencies. As the disease progresses, all frequencies are affected to some degree. Bone-conduction audiograms of patients with OTO typically show a greater loss at 2000 Hz—called a Carhart notch.[124] When OTO is limited to the stapedial footplate, a conductive hearing loss up to 65 dB may result. A loss greater than 65 dB would indicate that the cochlea has become involved.

## Management

A variety of treatments are available at each stage of the disease —amplification, surgery, and medication. But OTO presently has no cure.[125]

## Surgery

Primarily, the conductive form of OTO is treated surgically usually with stapedectomy. This procedure has several versions, most of which restore hearing when the disease is confined to the stapedial footplate and when cochlear function is normal.[126]

When OTO is conductive below 1000 Hz and sensorineural above 1000 Hz, surgery that reduces or eliminates the low-frequency component will not provide serviceable hearing and will make the patient a poorer candidate for amplification. Postoperatively, such patients will experience a drop in ability to discriminate speech in noise, a narrowed dynamic range, and the absence of a "cushioning" or dampening effect provided by the conductive component.[127]

When bone conduction is depressed by 30 to 35 dB across the frequency range but significantly better than air conduction, surgical intervention has less deleterious effect on speech recognition, but the patient still lacks serviceable hearing in many listening situations and requires amplification. In far-advanced forms of the disease—in which the joint between the stapedial footplate and the oval window is obliterated—aggressive drill-out surgery using microdrills to thin out the footplate creates an opening for a prosthesis.[128]

Once there is significant inner-ear involvement, surgery does not reverse the hearing loss and may not eliminate the tinnitus. Studies so far find that tinnitus is either relieved or eliminated in the majority of patients undergoing stapes surgery, but about 1 in 10 patients report that tinnitus remains the same or worsens postoperatively.[129]

## Amplification

If surgery is unsuccessful, hearing aids remain an option.[130] A mixed hearing loss complicates the choice between amplification and surgery. The conductive component tends to improve suprathreshold tolerance and to "flatten" the audiometric configuration, contributing to greater and earlier adjustment to amplification.

Hearing aids may vary in a patient's lifetime from completely in-the-canal hearing aids to powerful behind-the-ear instrumentation. Some patients have or continue to use conventional bone-conduction aids. Others become candidates for cochlear implants when their hearing losses become profound or total.

## *Medication*

Sodium fluoride has been prescribed to retard progression of the disease. It has fairly innocuous side effects, such as mottling of teeth, so it can be prescribed with impunity, especially in cases in which there is a rapid decline in bone conduction, but its use has aroused some controversy.[131-133]

## *Monitoring*

Annual audiologic examinations are recommended to check the disease's course and to provide benchmarks for treatment evaluation. Patients should be advised to have an evaluation when there is any subjective change in their hearing.

Periodic audiometry for family members of patients with OTO who do not seem affected by it appears justified by the likely genetic origin of the disorder. Such a precaution would ensure that intervention begins as early as possible, if subsequently found.

## PRESBYCUSIS

Presbycusis derives from the Greek *presbys* (old) and *kousis* (hearing), signifying the complex relationship between age and hearing loss.

## Frequency of Occurrence

It is the most frequently reported cause of hearing loss among older adults.[134,135]

A gender difference in the prevalence of this condition appears to favor females in the frequencies above 1000 Hz with superior retention of hearing in the low frequencies for males.[136] The overall severity of presbycusis is greater in males than females, which may result from (a) genetic factors and/or (b) greater exposure for males to high-intensity noise in work and recreation.[137]

## Etiology

The name seems to imply that hearing loss is a consequence of aging, as shown by the high correlation between age and hearing loss (Figure 1.3.1). Some studies challenge the notion that aging causes hearing loss.[138] Others assume the correlation indicates a genetic component because it appears to affect some persons and their parents and grandparents as early as the third decade of life and others retain excellent hearing (at least as measured by pure-tone sensitivity) into their eighth and ninth decades.[139] Many factors probably contribute to the hearing impairments found in the elderly; for example, prior infections, noise exposure, otosclerosis, and ototoxic drugs. Central auditory processing disorder (CAPD) may account for some "cognitive deficits." As people age, deterioration occurs at all levels of their auditory system.[140] Decrements in sensitivity, particularly for the higher frequencies, characterize much of the sensorineural hearing loss in the elderly.[141]

Although aging can affect any portion of the auditory system, presbycusis is viewed as involving primarily the cochlea and retrocochlear structures up to and including the CNS. Two additional forms of presbycusis have been identified: vascular presbycusis—resulting from deterioration of the blood supply to the lateral wall of the cochlear duct and the spiral lamina—and hyperosmotic presbycusis due to abnormal bone growth in the modiolus or internal auditory meatus compressing auditory nerve cells causing them to degenerate.[142,143]

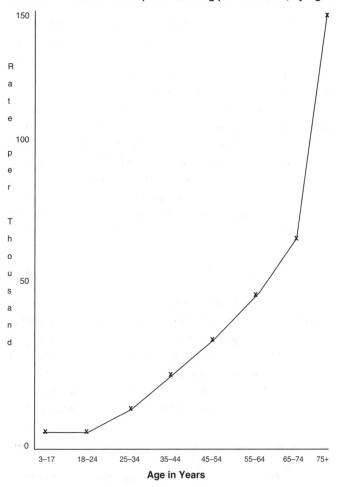

**Number of Persons with Impaired Hearing per Thousand, by Age**

*Rate per Thousand*

*Age in Years*

**Figure 1.3.1.** Number of persons with impaired hearing by age. From Ries PW. Prevalence and characteristics of persons with hearing trouble: United States, 1990-91. *Vital and Health Statistics.* 1994;Series 10(188):1

## Diagnosis

Most elderly persons enter their senior years with a lifetime of diseases, insults, and injuries to their auditory system. Although different types of presbycusis have been identified, the assertion that the types are accompanied by specific audiologic findings is often difficult to confirm audiometrically.[144,145]

Cognitive factors make necessary the inclusion in the initial audiologic evaluation of measures to detect CAPD. It may complicate diagnosis and management in some seniors who have greater difficulty hearing than would be expected from their audiograms.[146] Because CAPD is believed to affect up to three-fourths of the elderly population with hearing loss, testing for this condition should be required for all patients with presbycusis.[147]

## Management

Because of the gradual onset of presbycusis—possibly over several decades—elderly patients often come to rehabilitation reluctantly. They have been adapting to their hearing loss for so long they often tell clinicians, "I don't miss anything; it's just that people mumble." By the time elderly patients finally decide (or are driven by others) to seek help, the clinician will need patience convincing them that they are not too old to be helped.[148]

### *Amplification*

Real-ear measurements are used in the initial and postfitting visits.[149] Putting audiologic results in percentage terms rather than decibels can assist in convincing patients of their loss and its extent.

In recommending hearing aids, clinicians must be aware of elderly patients' possible physical limitations, like arthritis. They must have sufficient dexterity to change batteries, adjust volume controls, and properly insert ear molds and the hearing aid.

The greater the CNS involvement, the greater the time and effort required to derive benefit from amplification and the greater the need for expanded hearing rehabilitation often on an individual basis.

## Counseling

Counseling designed to address elderly patients' concerns about activities of daily living should be undertaken (also see Section 2.3). Repetition and reinforcement of instructions are essential. An empathic clinician is a more important determiner of success than the specific brand or style of hearing aid. Also important are arranging for a quiet place in which to talk with patients, because so many have difficulty understanding what is said against a noisy background.

Sending printed information home with patients can enable them to check with others, to ensure they have absorbed the information and instruction provided. The positive attitudes toward rehabilitation of family members and other significant persons can encourage patients to seek assistance and accept treatment.

The high correlation between aging and hearing loss arouses a dangerous attitude that may lead some elderly patients to accept as inevitable further damage to their hearing and to abandon hearing-conservation efforts. Instead, they need to be strongly urged to avoid prolonged, intense noise exposure and ototoxic drugs, to seek prompt treatment of ear infections, and to protect in all possible ways whatever hearing remains. Such counseling will enhance the hearing-aid use that has been prescribed by forestalling further hearing loss.

## Medication

A Dutch study provided evidence for slowing presbycusis by adding oral folic acid to the diets of older men and women. Although hearing continued to decline in the treated and untreated groups, the losses in the treated group's speech frequencies though statistically significant were clinically insignificant, pointing to the need for cross-validation.[150]

# STICKLER SYNDROME AND PIERRE-ROBIN SEQUENCE

Stickler syndrome (SS)—also known as Marshall-Stickler syndrome and Hereditary Arthro-Ophthalmopathy—consists of cleft palate, ocular defects (myopia, retinal detachment, cataracts), flattening of the facial profile, and arthropathy. SS is named after Gunnar B. Stickler, who described it in 1960.

SS has a closely related form designated Pierre-Robin sequence (PRS).[151] PRS symptoms typically comprise orofacial defects (cleft palate, unusually small lower jaw (micrognathia and glossoptosis) and otic anomalies (otitis media, auricular dysplasias, external auditory canal atresia, and conductive hearing loss). In addition to SS, PRS is related to Velocardiofacial syndrome, Möbius syndrome, and CHARGE association.

## Frequency of Occurrence

The incidence of SS is probably in the range of 1 to 3 per 10,000 births. PRS has been estimated at 1 per 8,500 live births, but the underlying estimate may include SS rather than being for PRS alone.[152] SS affects both genders.[153]

## Etiology

Although generally familial, the mode of inheritance of SS remains undetermined in some cases and open to question in others. A precise explanation of its relatively frequent concurrence with PRS lacks a consensus.

SS affects the connective tissues' collagen. Several genes that govern collagen synthesis may cause SS. As it is a progressive condition, not all aspects may appear at birth. The number of symptoms and the developmental time of their appearance depend on the genes involved: some may only cause the joint and hearing problems, whereas others give rise to different symptoms, as in Oto-spondylo-megaepiphyseal dysplasia.

In SS, hearing loss occurs in a sizable proportion of cases. The hearing loss is usually secondary to eustachian-tube malformations and palatal anomalies and is typically conductive.[154]

Independent of SS, PRS's etiology is heterogeneous. It has been considered, in different cases, to be an autosomal dominant and an autosomal recessive condition. Although PRS generally does not appear to favor males or females, an X-linked variation that includes clubfeet and heart problems has been reported. Three explanations have been advanced to account for PRS: mechanical, neurologic-maturation, and rhombencephalic anomaly. The mechanical explanation is most widely accepted.[155]

Cleft palate occurs in about 9 of 10 cases of SS. The potential ophthalmic disorders are myopia, a high risk of retinal detachments, cataracts and glaucoma, and conductive hearing loss.[156,157] Stiff and overly flexible joints, with late onset of osteoarthritis, also occur in about half the cases.

## Diagnosis

SS's symptoms and its severity are variable, making it somewhat difficult to diagnose. Differential diagnosis increases the difficulty because of its similarity to the several additional syndromes mentioned above. DNA analysis and familial history are essential to determining the cause(s) of SS and PRS.

Hearing losses often occur, so audiologic examination is essential, though not conclusive with respect to its etiology. Otitis media and auricular anomalies account for the major share of conductive hearing losses. A relatively small number of cases also have auditory-canal atresia and anomalies of the ossicles.[158]

## Management

Treatment begins with repair of the cleft palate, when present, and amplification, when there is a hearing loss. If middle-ear surgery to correct ossicular-chain defects does not yield serviceable hearing, amplification should be prescribed promptly.

Monitoring on an annual basis should be undertaken because there is a high risk of retinal detachment and late-onset hearing impairment. Early indications of such problems enable patients who experience any of SS's and PRS's numerous symptoms to seek appropriate care for them.

Treating the numerous features of SS and PRS requires a multidisciplinary team: audiologists, pediatricians, otolaryngologists, plastic surgeons, orthodontists, speech-language therapists, and social workers.[159] Referring the family to genetic counseling is recommended.

# TINNITUS

Tinnitus is a sensation of sound perceived in the absence of external stimuli. Patients localize it in one or both ears or "in the head." They describe it with a variety of adjectives, like "throbbing," "hissing," "ringing," or combinations of such sounds. These sensations are almost always subjective, but objective forms of tinnitus that are audible to others do occur, though rarely.

## Frequency of Occurrence

The American Tinnitus Association (ATA) estimates that 40 to 50 million persons in the United States experience tinnitus—a number that far exceeds the prevalence of hearing loss.[160] The number of people whose quality of life is adversely impacted by severe, intractable tinnitus is probably closer to 2.5 million.[161] Among U.S. veterans, 3 to 4 million report they have tinnitus, with up to one million of them seeking clinical intervention.[162] Although some prevalence estimates assume tinnitus may occur in the absence of hearing loss, an auditory basis for virtually all cases of significant tinnitus might be identified if given thorough audiologic evaluation.

About 80% of persons with chronic tinnitus say they are not overly annoyed by it. However, approximately 1 in 5 say it bothers them to the extent they require some form of relief.[163] For the latter persons, tinnitus can be a dominating force in their lives. Anxiety and depression are present in many of these individuals, and suicidal tendencies are not unusual.[164,165] Nearly one-fourth (669) of 2,800 older adults said tinnitus diminished their quality of life, referring to it in terms of physical pain and stress rather than mental or emotional effects.[166]

## Etiology

Like a headache or a cough, tinnitus is a symptom not a disease. Any otic or auditory disorder may give rise to tinnitus.

It is a significant early indicator of a hearing loss due to ototoxic medications or to an acoustic neuroma. Much inner-ear tinnitus also results from exposure to prolonged, intense noise levels.

When tinnitus arises from damage to the cochlea, it presents a more challenging condition—identified by air- and bone-conduction thresholds that are in close agreement, tests of word-recognition tests that reveal deficiencies, and measurements of otoacoustic emissions that indicate damage to the outer hair cells. In all such cases, tinnitus elimination typically cannot be achieved, and even its reduction is more difficult, although relief and some control may be obtained.

### *Objective Tinnitus*

Although the vast majority of cases of tinnitus are subjective, objective tinnitus heard by the patient and audible to others does occur. Some of the causes of objective tinnitus involve muscular, structural or vascular abnormalities. It has been observed in some degenerative diseases, like amyotrophic lateral sclerosis, causing a repetitive flutter of the middle-ear muscles and consequent mechanical sounds. It is even possible that elevated blood pressure and thyroid dysfunctions can cause objective tinnitus.[167]

## *Pulsatile Tinnitus*

Pulsatile tinnitus overlaps with the vascular pathologies causing objective tinnitus. Often unilateral, the condition may be the result of vascular pathology; for example, transmission of atrial or intratemporal carotid-artery pulsations. Even serous otitis media can give rise to this condition. Patients with pulsatile tinnitus need a comprehensive radiographic evaluation and consultation with an otologist skilled and experienced in managing patients with this and related conditions.[168]

## Diagnosis

The patient who presents with tinnitus requires thorough audiologic and otologic examinations. Because tinnitus may be present at frequencies not customarily tested in pure-tone audiometry, clinicians should use full-sweep Bekesy audiometry that tests all frequencies between 100 to 10,000 Hz and, with the necessary special equipment, above 10,000 Hz.

Audiologists should be cautious about testing the tinnitus patient's acoustic-reflex thresholds at high intensity because it might cause acoustic trauma or worsen the tinnitus. Likewise, clinicians should avoid measuring acoustic-reflex decay at 10 dB above the auditory-reflex threshold for the same reason.[169] When tinnitus accompanies asymmetrical and unilateral sensorineural hearing losses, auditory-brainstem testing and MRI should be performed before considering tinnitus management, to rule out auditory tumors and other pathology.[170]

## *Tinnitus Inventories*

A tinnitus questionnaire and a stress inventory should be administered to all patients with the complaint of tinnitus. Upon their completion, the clinician reviews their responses and discusses treatment options with them in a relaxed, supportive environment. Among such instruments, the Tinnitus Handicap Inventory has been subjected to statistical analysis and provides encouraging evidence for its validity.[171,172]

## Management

Management of tinnitus falls into three categories: direct intervention to eliminate or ameliorate it, masking to overcome its effects, and education to assist in the process of adaptation to it.[173]

### *Direct Intervention*

Some treatments may relieve or even eliminate tinnitus; for example, removal of impacted cerumen or excision of an acoustic tumor. When such procedures are successful, the tinnitus often abates or ceases altogether.

### *Hearing Aids*

Instrumentation, such as maskers and hearing aids, are virtually free of any side effects, when they are professionally prescribed and monitored. Clinicians who instruct their patients in the use of these instruments provide the added advantage of giving patients a means by which they can react positively to tinnitus; that is, they can cease to be its victims and are empowered to exert a degree of control over an unwelcome visitor.

The patient whose tinnitus occurs in the range above 1000 Hz should be evaluated for hearing-aid use. Hearing aids can facilitate the intermittent suppression of tinnitus after auditory stimulation (residual inhibition). It may also direct patients' attention away from their tinnitus.[174]

Fitting hearing aids for the tinnitus sufferer with minimal high-frequency hearing loss may be recommended even when, without the tinnitus, the use of amplification would not be advised.

To gain full benefit from instruments that contain both a masker and an amplification circuit, clinicians should guide their use and they should include a volume control that enables the patient to have some control over their tinnitus.

Phase-shift treatment uses sound cancellation to induce partial or complete inhibition to the frequency of the patient's tinnitus for an extended period of time.[175] A study of 61 patients with tinnitus found a high correlation between treatment and decrease in tinnitus intensity.[176] A Swedish study reported similarly favorable results.[177]

Periodic monitoring of hearing status while hearing aids or maskers are in use is essential.

## *Masking*

For some tinnitus sufferers, masking provides relief. To aid sleep, for example, a speaker placed under the pillow connected to a sound source plays throughout the night. During waking hours, wearable maskers that provide sound to counter the tinnitus may be prescribed.[178,179]

The maskability of the patient's tinnitus needs to be determined by having patients match their tinnitus to an audiometric frequency or frequencies and determining its loudness. The clinician then presents the patient with a narrow band of noise centered at the frequency of the tinnitus for one minute via earphones at a level rendering the patient's tinnitus inaudible. When the masking noise is removed, the clinician asks the patient whether the tinnitus has become better, worse, unchanged, or different in quality. The presence of residual inhibition is considered a favorable indicator for the use of masking.[180]

Patients with cochlear implants sometimes report it improved or eliminated their tinnitus. Successful stapedectomy for otosclerosis also may affect tinnitus.[181,182] Exceptions have been noted in which tinnitus remains the same or worsens after surgery or is noticed more in the nonoperated ear.[183]

## *Tinnitus Retraining Therapy (TRT)*

TRT also known as habituation or desensitization therapy has become an increasingly popular method of treating severe, intractable tinnitus.[184] Although a tinnitus masker is used, the level of the masking is below the point at which the tinnitus is obscured. Instead, patients are repeatedly exposed to audible signals from the masker and their own tinnitus in a controlled, supportive setting.[185]

TRT is reported to be successful in over 70% of such patients. However, it is unclear how much of the improvement is a result of habituation and how much is the result of the intensive one-on-one counseling, which is a critical component of the therapy and which takes most patients 18 months before success is realized. Long-term follow-up is essential to determine TRT's efficacy, as it is in all forms of tinnitus therapy.[186]

## *Cognitive Rehabilitation Therapy (CRT)*

CRT aims to correct the patient's misperceptions about their tinnitus. Adapted from a treatment for depression, it is short-term and involves a contract with the tinnitus patient. The clinician addresses these maladaptive cognitions in terms of scientific data relevant to patients' concerns and appropriate to their educational levels and coping mechanisms.[187,188]

A study of groups receiving education only, education combined with CRT, and a no-treatment waiting list found no significant benefit for the control group.[189] Another study found reduced self-perceived tinnitus impairment following a single group session.[190] When group counseling based on TRT principles was combined with masking, it provided statistically more benefit than either traditional support or no treatment.[191]

## *Neuromonics Tinnitus Treatment (NTT)*

NTT was formerly called Acoustic Desensitization Protocol. It combines acoustic stimulation with a program of counseling and support. The acoustic component provides stimulation to auditory pathways and to the limbic system that is presumed to be deprived by hearing loss. Intermittently associating the tinnitus with pleasant, relaxing sound desensitizes the patient's reactions to the tinnitus. Patients are provided with a personal sound player and a recording matched to their audiometric profiles.[192]

NTT has received FDA clearance. A study reported that 32 of 35 subjects with moderate to severe tinnitus attained relief.[193]

## Medication

Numerous medications, herbal extracts, and vitamins have been prescribed for tinnitus relief. Most have not had scientific studies and, when studied, have not been shown to be effective. As for positive anecdotal accounts, the powerful placebo effect provides a likely explanation of such positive results. When these agents seem to work, they probably relieve the anxiety and/or depression rather than the tinnitus.[194,195]

Melatonin supplementation showed a statistically, but not clinically, significant decrease in their scores on the Tinnitus Handicap Inventory.[196] These results may encourage studies with larger doses and, perhaps, over longer periods.[197]

A double-blind, randomized study of the herbal remedy *Ginko biloba* found no significant differences in tinnitus alleviation between the 478 placebo and treatment pairs.[198] As with studies of Melatonin, further research using higher dosages of *Ginko biloba* over a longer time might obtain results favoring it. Such investigations are underway.[199]

One medication that may provide relief from tinnitus is Xanax (Alprazolam). A double-blind study showed 76% of the treated subjects experienced a reduction of tinnitus, whereas only 5% of the placebo subjects reported improvement.[200]

## Other Therapies and Lifestyle Modification

Among the other treatments that have been suggested are acupuncture, biofeedback training, transcutaneous nerve stimulation, craniocervical massage, and various forms of relaxation therapy. Most of these techniques have not been subjected to systematic study, and reports of success are based primarily on anecdotal reports.[201]

A comprehensive, integrated approach to tinnitus control and management focuses on the overall emotional well-being of the patient, using management and coping strategies. It postulates a common genetic cause of tinnitus and depression—possibly the serotonin transporter gene SLC6A4—and includes informational counseling, sound therapy, and other management strategies.[202]

Clinicians recommend that tinnitus sufferers avoid alcohol, aspirin, caffeine, tobacco, and ototoxic drugs, such as aminoglycosides. Persons at risk should advise their physicians of their vulnerability, seek their advice with respect to any less ototoxic treatments, and report the onset of tinnitus and any changes in their hearing when initiating a new medication.[203]

## *Surgery*

In several degenerative diseases of the head and neck, loss of control of the tensor tympani or stapedius muscle occurs, causing tinnitus that can be surgically relieved. A dentist specializing in the treatment of temperomandibular joint (TMJ) syndrome can provide relief from tinnitus that often accompanies TMJ.[204]

## *Monitoring*

Audiologic monitoring on a regular basis is essential for all patients fitted with maskers, hearing aids, or a combination instrument. Even those who choose no treatment should be followed to detect significant alterations in hearing and/or tinnitus and to continue to provide counseling.[205]

## **REFERENCES**

1. Alpert syndrome. Retrieved May 2007 from http://www. biology-online.org/dictionary/alpert_syndrome.

2. Michel P. Memoire sur les anomalies congenitales de l'oreille interne. *Gazette Med Strasbourg*. 1863;23:55-58.

3. Jackler RK, Luxford WM, House WF. Congenital malformations of the inner ear: a classification based on embryogenesis. *Laryngoscope*. 1987;97(suppl 40):2-14.

4. Strome SE, Baker KB, Langman AW. Imaging case of the month: inner ear malformation. *Am J Otol*. 1998;19:396-397.

5. Rapin I. Conductive hearing loss effects on children's language and scholastic skills. A review of the literature. *Ann Otol Rhinol Laryngol*. 1979;88:3-12.

6. Phillips DP. An introduction to auditory neuroscience. In: Musiek FE, Chermak GD, eds. *Handbook of (Central) Auditory Disorder: Auditory Neuroscience and Diagnosis*. Vol 1. San Diego, Calif: Plural Publishing; 2007.

7. National Institute of Deafness and Other Communicative Disorders. Access at http://www.nidcd.nih.gov

8. Bamiou D, Musiek F, Luxon L. Aetiology and clinical processing disorders: a review. *Arch Dis Childh*. 2001;85:361-365.

9. Baron JA, Musiek FE. Behavioral assessment of the central auditory nervous system. In: Musiek FE, Rintlemann WF eds. *Contemporary Prospectives in Hearing Assessment*. Boston, Mass: Allyn & Bacon; 1999.

10. Jerger J, Musiek F. Report of the Consensus Conference on the Diagnosis of Auditory Processing Disorders in School-Aged Children. *J Am Acad Audiol*. 2000;11(9):467-474.

11. Keith RW, Novak KK. Relationships between tests of central auditory function and receptive language. *Sem Hear*. 1984;5:243-250.

12. Stach BA. *Clinical Audiology: An Introduction*. San Diego, Calif: Singular; 1998.

13. Kids Health. Retreived September 2007 from http://www.kidshealth.org

14. American Speech-Language-Hearing Association. *Auditory Integration Training* [Technical Report]. Retrieved 2004 from http://www.asha.org/docs/html/TR2004-00260.html

15. American Speech-Language-Hearing Association. *Auditory Integration Training* [Position Statement]. Retrieved 2004 from http://www.asha.org/docs/html/PS2004-00218.html

16. Starr A, Picton TW, Sininger Y, et al. Auditory neuropathy. *Brain*. 1996;119:741-753.

17. Rapin I, Gravel JS. A biologically inappropriate label unless acoustic nerve involvement is documented. *J Am Acad Audiol.* 2006;17:147–150.

18. Audiology awareness campaign: auditory neuropathy and auditory dyssychrony. Retrieved 2007 from http://www.audi ologyawareness.com

19. Stein L, Tremblay K, Pasternak J, et al. Brainstem abnormalities in neonates with normal otoacoustic emissions. *Sem Hearing.* 1996;17:197–213.

20. Sininger Y, Hood L, Starr A, et al. Hearing loss due to auditory neuropathy. *Audiology.* 1995;7:11–13.

21. Hood LJ. Auditory neuropathy. What is it and what can we do about it? *Hear J.* 1998;51:10–18.

22. Lanarz T, Lim HH, Reuter G, et al. The auditory midbrain implant: a new auditory prosthesis for neural deafness—concept and device description. *Otol Neurotol.* 2006;27: 838–843.

23. Colletti V, Fiorino FG, Carner M, et al. Auditory brainstem implant as a salvage treatment after unsuccessful cochlear implantation. *Otol Neurotol.* 2004;25:485–496.

24. McCabe B. Autoimmune sensorineural hearing loss. *Ann Otorhinolaryngol.* 1979;88:314–322.

25. National Institute of Allergy and Infectious Diseases. Retrieved May 2006 from http://www.niaid.gov

26. DiGiovanni JJ, Nair P. Spontaneous recovery of sudden sensorineural hearing loss: possible association with autoimmune disorders. *J Am Acad Audiol.* 2006;17(7): 498–505.

27. Martin JL, Mestril R, Hilal-Dandan R, et al. Small heat shock proteins and protection against ischemic injury in cardiac myocytes. *Circulation.* 1997;96:4343–4348.

28. Sismanis A, Thompson T, Willis HE. Methotrexate management of immune-mediated cochleovestibular disorders. *Laryngoscope.* 1994;104:932–934.

29. Sismanis A, Wise CM, Johnson GI. Methotrexate management of immune-mediated cochleovestibular disorders. *Otorhinolaryngol Head Neck Surg.* 1997;116:146–152.

30. Horn CE, Himel HN, Selesnick SH. Hyperbaric oxygen therapy for sudden sensorineural hearing loss: a prospective trial of patients failing steroid and antiviral treatment. *Otol Neurotol.* 2005;26(5):878–881.

31. Huy PTB, Sauvaget E. Idiopathic Sudden sensorineural hearing loss is not an otologic emergency. *Otol Neurotol.* 2005; 26(5):896–902.

32. Sweetow RW, Robert KW, Philliposian C. Considerations for cochlear implantation in children with sudden fluctuating hearing loss. *J Am Acad Audiol.* 2005;16:770–780.

33. Toricella H. CHARGE association. *J Am Acad Audiol.* 1995; 6(1):47–53.

34. Lin AE, Siebent JR, Graham JM. CNS malformations in the CHARGE association. *Am J Med Genet.* 1990;37:304–310.

35. Davenport SL, Hefner MA, Thelin JW. CHARGE syndrome. Part I, External ear anomalies. *Int J Pediatr Otorhinolaryngol.* 1986;12:137–143.

36. Wiener-Vacher SR, Denise P, Narcey P, et al. Vestibular function in children with the CHARGE association. *Arch Otolaryngol Head Neck Surg.* 1999;125:342–34.

37. Northern JL, Downs MP. *Hearing in Children.* 5th ed. Baltimore, Md: Lippincott Williams & Wilkins; 2002.

38. Blake KD, Russell-Eggitt IM, Morgan DW, et al. Who's in CHARGE? Multidisciplinary management of patients with CHARGE association. *Arch Dis Childh.* 1990;65(2):217–223.

39. Edwards BM, Kileny PR, Van Riper LA. CHARGE syndrome: A window of opportunity for audiologic intervention. *Pediatrics.* 2002;110(1):119–126.

40. Chang EH, Van Camp G, Smith RJ. The role of connexins in human disease. *Ear Hear.* 2003;24:314–323.

41. Nance WE, Kearsey MJ. Relevance of connexin in deafness (DFNB1) to human evolution. *Am J Hum Genet.* 2004;74(6): 1091–1087.

42. Abe S, Usami S, Shinkawa H, et al. Prevalent connexin 26 gene (GJB2) mutations in Japanese. *J Med Genet.* 2000;37:41–43.

43. Wiszniewski W, Sobieszczanska-Radoszewska L, Nowakowska-Szyrwinska E, et al. High frequency of GJB2 gene mutations in Polish patients with prelingual nonsyndromic deafness. *Genet Test.* 2001;5(2):147–148.

44. Oliveira CA, Maciel-Guerra AT, Sartorato EL. Deafness resulting from mutations in the GJB2 (connexin 26) gene in Brazilian patients. *Clin Gene.* 2002;61(5):354–358.

45. Kikuchi T, Kimura RS, Paul DL, et al. Gap junction systems in

the mammalian cochlea. *Brain Res Brain Res Rev*. 2000;32: 163–166.

46. Zhang Y, Tang W, Ahmad S, et al. Gap-junction-mediated intercellular biochemical coupling in cochlear supporting cells is required for normal cochlear functions. *Proc Nat Acad Sci U.S.A.* 2005;102:15201–15206.

47. Thonnissen E, Rabionet R, Arbones ML, et al. Human connexin 26 (GJB2) deafness mutations affect the function of gap junction channels at different levels of protein expression. *Hum Genet*. 2002;111:190–197.

48. Stong BC, Chang Q, Ahmad S, et al. A novel mechanism for Connexin 26 mutation linked deafness: cell death caused by leaky gap junction hemichannels. *Laryngoscope*. 2006;116: 2205–2210.

49. Liang GS, de Miguel M, Gomez-Hernandez JM, et al. Severe neuropathy with leaky connexin 32 hemichannels. *Ann Neurol*. 2005;57:749–754.

50. Manthey D, Willecke K. Transfection and expression of exogenous connexins in mammalian cells. In: Bruzzone R, Giaume C, eds. *Connexin Methods and Protocols*. Totowa, NJ: Humana Press; 2001.

51. Prasad S, Cucci RA, Green GE, et al. Genetic testing for hereditary hearing loss: connexin 26 (GJB2) allele variants and two novel deafness-causing mutations (R32C and 645-648delT-AGA). *Hum Mutations*. 2000;16:502–508.

52. Beltramello M, Piazza V, Bukauskas FF, et al. Impaired permeability to Ins(1,4,5)P(3) in a mutant connexin underlies recessive hereditary deafness. *Nature Cell Biol*. 2005;7:63–69.

53. Selikowitz M. *Down Syndrome: The Facts*. New York, NY: Oxford University Press; 1990.

54. Down JLH. Observations on an ethnic classification of idiots. *Clinical Lectures and Reports by the Medical and Surgical Staff of the London Hospital*. 1866;3:259–262.

55. Horoupian D. Pathology of the central auditory pathways and cochlear nerve. In: Alberti PW, Ruben RJ, eds. *Otologic Medicine and Surgery*. New York, NY: Churchill Livingstone; 1988.

56. O'Leary VB, Parie-McDermott A, Molloy AM, et al. MTRR and MTHFR Polymorphism: link to Down Syndrome? *Am J Med Genet*. 2002;107(2):151–155.

57. American College of Obstetricians and Gynecologists (ACOG). Screening for fetal chromosomal Abnormalities. *ACOG Practice Bull.* 2007;77:1–14.

58. Sando I, Haruo T. Otitis media in association with various congenital diseases. *Ann Otol Rhinol Laryngol.* 1990;5148:13–16.

59. Aase JM, Wilson AC, Smith DW. Small ears in Down's syndrome: a helpful diagnostic aid. *J Pediatrics.* 1973;82:845–847.

60. Balkany TJ, Mischke RE, Downs MP, et al. Ossicular abnormalities in Down's syndrome. *Otol Head Neck Surg.* 1979;87: 372:384.

61. Maroudias N, Economides J, Christodoulov P, et al. A study on the otoscopical and audiological findings in patients with Down's syndrome in Greece. *Int J Pediatr Otorhinolaryngol.* 1984;29:43–49.

62. Bilgin H, Kasemsuwan S, Schachern PA, et al. Temporal bone study of Down's syndrome. *Otol Head Neck Surg.* 1996;122: 271–275.

63. Keiser H, Montague J, Wold D, et al. Hearing loss in Down's syndrome adults. *Am J Ment Def.* 1981;85(5):467–472.

64. Walford RL. Immunology and aging. *Am J Clin Pathol.* 1980; 74:247–253.

65. Turner S, Sloper P, Cunningham C, et al. Health problems in children with Down's syndrome. *Child Care Hlth Develop.* 1990;16:83–97.

66. American Academy of Pediatrics Committee on Genetics. Health Supervision for Children with Down Syndrome. *Pediatrics.* 2001;107(2): 442–449.

67. March of Dimes. Retrieved August 2007 from http://www. marchofdimes.com/professionals/14332_1214.asp

68. Wynne, MK, Diefendorf AO, Fritsch MH. Sudden hearing loss. *Asha Leader.* 2001;6(23):6–8.

69. Meyerhoff WL, Paparella MM. Medical therapy for sudden deafness. In: Snow JB, ed. *Controversy in Otolaryngology.* Philadelphia, Pa: WB Saunders; 1980.

70. Wazen JJ, Ghossaini SN. The diagnostic and treatment dilemma of sudden sensorineural hearing loss. *Hear Rev.* 2003;10(13):38,40,41.

71. Chen C, Halpin C, Rauch SD. Oral steroid therapy for sudden sensorineural hearing loss in a ten-year retrospective analysis. *Otol Neurol.* 2003;24:728–733.

72. Sano H, Okamoto M, Shitara T, et al. What kind of patients are suitable for evaluating the therapeutic effect of sudden deafness? *Am J Otol*. 1998;19:579-583.

73. Wazen JJ, Spitzer JB, Ghossaini SN, et al. Transcranial contralateral cochlear stimulation in unilateral deafness. *Otol Head Neck Surg*. 2003;129(3):248-254.

74. Yanagita N, Murahashi K. Bilateral simultaneous sudden deafness. *Arch Otorhinolaryngol*. 1987;244:7-10.

75. Ohta F. Simultaneous bilateral sudden deafness. *Audiol Japan*. 1970;13:138-143.

76. Lee H, Whitman GT, Lim JG. Bilateral sudden deafness as a prodrome of anterior inferior cerebellar artery infarction. *Arch Neurol*. 2001;58:1287-1289.

77. Oh J-H, Park K, Lee SJ, et al. Bilateral versus unilateral sudden sensorineural hearing loss. *Otol Head Neck Surg*. 2007;136: 87-91.

78. Fayad JN, Delacruz A. Etiologies and treatment options for sudden sensorineural hearing loss. *Hear Rev*. 2003;10(13):20-23.

79. Byl FM. Sudden hearing loss: eight years' experience and suggested prognostic table. *Laryngoscope*. 1984;94:647-661.

80. Halpin C, Rauch S. Steroid therapy for sudden sensorineural hearing loss. *Hear Rev*. 2003;32:34-35.

81. Nageris BI, Ulanovski D, Attias J. Magnesium treatment for sudden hearing loss. *Ann Otol Rhinol Laryngol*. 2004;113: 672-675.

82. Joachims HZ, Segal J, Golz A, et al. Antioxidants in treatment of idiopathic sudden hearing loss. *Otol Neurotol*. 2003;24(4): 572-575.

83. Conlin AE, Parnes LS. Treatment of sudden sensorineural hearing loss. A systematic review. *Arch Otolaryngol Head Neck Surg*. 2007;133:573-574.

84. Sullivan RF. Transcranial ITE CROS. *Hear Instr*. 1988;39(1): 11-12, 54.

85. Harford E, Dodds E. The clinical application of CROS—a hearing aid for unilateral deafness. *Arch Otol Head Neck Surg*. 1966;83:73-82.

86. Valente M. Fitting options for unilateral hearing loss. *Hear J*. 1995;48:45-48.

87. Wazen JJ, Spitzer JB, Kuller M. Localization by unilateral BAHA users. *Otol Head Neck Surg*. 2005;132:928-932.

88. Schein JD, Miller MH. Sudden deafness: an auditory mystery. *Hear Hlth.* 1999;16(4):16–18.

89. Centers for Disease Control. Retrieved May 2007 from http://www.cdc.gov

90. Hall JW, Mueller HG. *Audiologists' Desk Reference.* Vol 1. San Diego, Calif: Singular; 1998.

91. Wladislavosky WP, Facer JW, Bahram M, et al. A 30-year epidemiologic and clinical study in Rochester, Minn 1951–1980. *Laryngoscope.* 1983;94:1217–1221.

92. Gelfand SA. Sudden Deafness. In: Gelfand SA, ed. *Essentials of Audiology.* 2nd ed. New York, NY: Thieme; 2001.

93. Kagan A, Hood JD. Neurological manifestations of migraine. *Brain.* 1984;107:1123–1142.

94. Gantz BJ, Samy RN. Meniere's disease. In: Rakel RE, Bope ET, eds. *Conn's Current Therapy.* Philadelphia, Pa: WB Saunders Company; 2002:917–919.

95. Dornhoffer JL, Danner C, Zhou L, et al. Atrial natriuretic peptide receptor upregulation in the rat inner ear. *Ann Otol Rhinol Laryngol.* 2002;3:1040–1044.

96. Quortrup K, Rostgaard J, Holstein-Rathlov N-H. The inner ear produces a natriuretic hormone. *Am J Physiol.* 1996;170:1073–1077.

97. Ferraro JA, Durrant JD. Electrocochleography in the evaluation of patients with Meniere's disease/endolymphatic hydrops. *J Am Acad Audiol.* 2006;17:45–68.

98. Jacobson JT. Short-latency auditory evoked potentials. In: Northern JL, ed. *Hearing Disorders.* 3rd ed. Boston, Mass: Allyn & Bacon; 1996.

99. Radke A, Lempert T, Gresty MA, et al. Migraine and Meniere's disease. Is there a link? *Neurology.* 2002;59:1700–1704.

100. Hinchcliff R. Headache and Meniere's disease. *Acta Otolaryngol.* 1967;63:384–390.

101. Kagan A, Hood JD. Neurological manifestations of migraine. *Brain.* 1984;107:1123–1142.

102. Shepard NT. Differentiation of Meniere's disease and migraine-associated dizziness. *J Am Acad Audiol.* 2006;17:69–80.

103. Brockwell CW, Bojrab DI. Background and technique of rotational testing. In: Jacobson GP, Newman CP, Kartush JM,

eds. *Handbook of Balance Function Testing*. St. Louis, Mo: Mosby; 1993.

104. Yellin MW, Mainord JC. *Evaluation of the Dizzy Patient: The package*. Instructional course presented at the American Academy of Audiology, Salt Lake City, Utah; 1996.

105. Furman JM, Marcus DA, Balaban CD. Migrainous vertigo: development of a pathogenic model and structured diagnostic interview. *Curr Opin Neurol*. 2003;16:5–13.

106. Pulec JL. Meniere's disease. In: Northern JL, ed. *Hearing Disorders*. 3rd ed. Boston, Mass: Allyn & Bacon; 1996.

107. Tuse RV. Diagnosis and management of neuro-otological disorders due to migraine. In: Herdman SJ, ed. *Vestibular Rehabilitation*. Philadelphia, Pa: FA Davis; 2000.

108. Hamill TA. Evaluating treatments for Meniere's disease: controversies surrounding placebo control. *J Am Acad Audiol*. 2006;17:27–37.

109. Morrison AW. The surgery of vertigo: saccus drainage for idiopathic endolymphatic hydrops. *J Laryngol Otol*. 1976;90: 87–93.

110. Bretlau P, Thomsen J, Tos M, et al. Placebo effect in surgery for Meniere's disease: a three-year follow-up study of patients in a double-blind placebo-controlled study on endolymphatic sac shunt surgery. *Am J Otol*. 1984;5(6):558–562.

111. Ghossaini SN, Wazen JJ. An update on the surgical treatment of Meniere's diseases. *J Am Acad Audiol*. 2006;17:38–44.

112. Lange G, Maurer J, Mann W. Long-term results after interval therapy with intratympanic gentamycin for Meniere's disease. *Laryngoscope*. 2004;114:102–105.

113. Perez N, Martin E, Zubieta JL, et al. BPPV in patients with Meniere's disease treated with intratympanic gentamycin. *Laryngoscope*. 2002;112:1104–1109.

114. Gates GA. Meniere's disease review 2005. *J Am Acad Audiol*. 2006;17:16–26.

115. Gates GA, Green JD Jr, Tucci DL, et al. The effects of transtympanic micro-pressure treatment in people with unilateral Meniere's disease. *Arch Otolaryngol Head Neck Surg*. 2004; 130:718–725.

116. Politzer A. *Diseases of the Ear*. 5th ed. London, UK: Bailliere; 1909.

117. Otosclerosis. Retrieved September 2007 from http://www.boystownhospital.org/Hearing/info/genetics/syndromes/otos.asp

118. Niedermeyer HP, Neubert WJ, Sedlmeier R. Persistent measles virus infection as a possible cause of otosclerosis; state of the art. *ENT J.* 2000;79(8):522-556, 558.

119. Gristwood RE. Otosclerosis (otospongiosis): general considerations. In: Alberti PW, Ruben RJ, eds. *Otologic Medicine and Surgery*. New York, NY: Churchill-Livingston; 1988.

120. Schaap T, Gapany-Gapanavicius B. The genetics of otosclerosis. I. Distorted sex ratio. *Am J Hum Genet.* 1978;1:59-64.

121. Derlacki EL. Otosclerosis. In: JL Northern, ed. *Hearing Disorders*. 3rd ed. Boston, Mass: Allyn & Bacon; 1996.

122. Bachor E, Wright JT, Pan HWP, Karmody CS. Fixation of the stapes footplate in children: a clinical and temporal bone histologic study. *Otol Neurotol.* 2005;26(5):866-873.

123. Booth J. Otosclerosis. *Practitioner.* 1978;221:710.

124. Carhart R. Clinical applications of bone conduction. *Arch Otolaryngol.* 1950;51:798-807.

125. Dinces EA, Wiet RJ. Medical and surgical management of middle ear disease. In: Valente M, Hosford-Dunn H, Roeser RJ, eds. *Audiology Treatment*. New York, NY: Thieme; 2000:338-339.

126. House HP, Hansen MR, Al Dakhail AA, et al. Stapedectomy versus stapedotomy: comparison of results with long-term follow-up. *Laryngoscope.* 2002;112(11):2046-2050.

127. Del Bo M, Zaghis A, Ambrosetti V. Some observations concerning 200 stapedectomies: fifteen years postoperatively. *Laryngoscope.* 1987;97:1211-1213.

128. Eviatar A. Stapes surgery. In: Alberti PW, Ruben RJ, eds. *Otologic Medicine and Surgery*. New York, NY: Churchill-Livingston; 1988.

129. Szymanski M, Golabek W, Mills R. Effect of stapedectomy on subjective tinnitus. *J Laryngol Otol.* 2003;117:261-264.

130. Meyerhoff WH, Marple BF, Roland PS. Tympanic membrane, middle ear and mastoid. In: Roland PS, Marple BF, Meyerhoff WL, eds. *Hearing Loss*. New York, NY: Thieme; 1997.

131. Colletti V, Fiorino FG. Effect of sodium fluoride on early stages of otosclerosis. *Am J Otol.* 1991;12(3):195-198.

132. Causse JR, Chevance LG, Shambaugh GE. Clinical experience and experimental findings with sodium fluoride in otosclero-

sis (otospongiosis). *Ann Otol Rhinol Laryngol.* 1974;83: 643–647.

133. Bretlau P, Salomon G, Johnsen NJ. Otospongiosis and sodium fluoride. A clinical double-blind, placebo-controlled study on sodium fluoride treatment in otospongiosis. *Am J Otol.* 1989;10(1):20–22.

134. Stach BA. *Clinical Audiology: An Introduction.* San Diego, Calif: Singular; 1998.

135. Newby HA. *Audiology.* 4th ed. Englewood Cliffs, NJ: Prentice-Hall; 1979:89.

136. Weinstein BE. *Geriatric Audiology.* New York, NY: Thieme; 2000.

137. Ward WD, Royster JD, Royster LH. Auditory and non-auditory effects of noise. In: Berger EH, Royster LH, Royster JD, et al. eds. *The Noise Manual.* 5th ed. Fairfax, Va: American Industrial Hygiene Association; 2000.

138. Rosen S, Bergman M, Dietrich P, et al. Presbycusis study of relatively noise-free population in the Sudan. *Ann Otol Rhinol Laryngol.* 1962;71:727–743.

139. Schein JD. Implications of hearing loss in the elderly population. *Hear Rehab Quart.* 1985;10(3):3–7.

140. Lebo CP, Redell RC. The presbycusis component in occupational hearing loss. *Laryngoscope.* 1972;83:1399–1409.

141. Bellis TJ. Differential diagnosis of (central) auditory processing in older listeners. In: Chermak GD, Musiek FE, eds. *Handbook of (Central) Auditory Processing Disorders. Vol I.* San Diego, Calif: Plural; 2006.

142. Johnsson LG. Vascular changes in the human inner ear. *Adv Otorhinolaryngol.* 1973;20:197–220.

143. Krmpotic-Nemanic J., Nemanic D, Kostovic I. Macroscopical and microscopical changes in the bottom of the internal auditory meatus. *Acta Otolaryngol.* 1972;73:254–258.

144. Schuknecht HF. Presbycusis. *Laryngoscope.* 1955;65:402.

145. Gelfand SA, ed. *Essentials of Audiology.* 2nd ed. New York, NY: Thieme; 2001.

146. Martin JS, Jerger JF. Some effects of aging on auditory processing. *J Rehab Res Develop.* 2006;42(4):25.

147. Bellis TJ. Auditory processing disorders: It's not just kids who have them. *Hear J.* 2003;56(5):10–20.

148. Kricos PB, Lesner SA. Hearing care for the older adult: *Audiologic Rehabilitation*. Boston, Mass: Butterworth-Heinemann; 1995.

149. Scollie S, Seewald R. Hearing aid fitting and verification procedures for children. In: Katz J, ed, *Handbook of Clinical Audiology*. 5th ed. New York, NY: Lippincott Williams & Wilkins, 2002:698–703.

150. Durga J, Verhoef P, Antenuis JC, et al. Effects of folic acid supplementation on hearing in older adults. *Ann Internal Med*. 2007;146:1–9.

151. Soulier M, Sigaudy S, Chau C, et al. Prenatal diagnosis of Pierre-Robin sequence as part of Stickler syndrome. *Prenat Diag*. 2002;22(7):567–568.

152. Elliott MA, Studen-Pavlovich DA, Ranalli DN. Prevalence of selected pediatric conditions in children with Pierre Robin sequence. *Pediatr Dent*. 1995;17(2):106–111.

153. Khan SY, Paul R, Sengupta A, et al. Clinical study of otological manifestations in cases of cleft palate. *Indian J Otol Head Neck Surg*. 2006;58:35–37.

154. Castillo MP, Roland PS. Disorders of the auditory system. In: Roeser RJ, Valente M, Hosford-Dunn H, eds. *Audiologic Diagnosis*. New York, NY: Thieme; 2000.

155. Dionisopoulos T, Williams HB. *Congenital Anomalies of the Ear, Nose and Throat*. New York, NY: Oxford University Press; 1997.

156. Fria TJ, Paradise JL, Sabo DL et al. Conductive hearing loss in children with cleft palate. *J Pediatrics*. 1987;3:84–87.

157. Franz N, Scheuerla J, Bequer N. Middle ear tissue mass in audiometric data from otologic care of infants with cleft palate. *Cleft Palate J*. 1988;25:170–171.

158. Gruen PM, Carranza A, Karmody CS, et al. Anomalies of the ear in the Pierre Robin triad. *Ann Otol Rhinol Laryngol*. 2005;114(8):605–613.

159. Bath AP, Bull PD. Management of upper airway obstruction in Pierre Robin sequence. *J Laryngol Otol*. 1997;111(12):1155–1157.

160. Henry JA, Jastreboff MM, Jastreboff PJ, et al. 2002. Assessment of patients for treatment with tinnitus retraining therapy. *J Am Acad Audiol*. 2000; 13:523–544.

161. Davis A, Refaie AE. Epidemiology of tinnitus. In: Tyler R, ed. *Tinnitus Handbook*. San Diego, Calif: Singular; 2000:1–23.

162. Henry JA, Schechter MA, Regelein RI, et al. Veterans and tinnitus. In: Snow JB, ed. *Tinnitus: Theory and Management*. Lewiston, NY: BC Decker; 2004.

163. Dobie RA. 2004. Overview: suffering from tinnitus. In: Snow JB, ed. *Tinnitus: Theory and Management*. Lewiston, NY: BC Decker; 2004.

164. Miller MH, Crane MA, Fox J. Intractable tinnitus: Managing the psychological component. *Am Audiol Soc Bull*. 1995;20:2.

165. Beck AT, Steer RA, Brown G, et al. Dysfunctional attitudes and suicidal ideation in psychiatric outpatients. *Suicide Life Threat Behav*. 1993;23:1,11–20.

166. Nordahl D, Cruickshanks KJ, Dalton DS, et al. The impact of tinnitus on quality of life in older adults. *J Am Acad Audiol*. 2000;18(3):257–286.

167. Rizer FM. *Inner ear and tinnitus*. Retrieved December 2004 from http://emedicine.com/ent/topic.235.htm

168. Tucci DL, Gray L. Radiographic imaging in otologic disease. In: Roeser RJ, Valente M, Hosford-Dunn H, eds. *Audiologic Diagnosis*. New York, NY: Thieme; 2000.

169. Miller, MH, Hoffman RA, Smallberg G. Stapedial reflex testing and partially reversible acoustic trauma. *Hear Instr*. 1984; 36(6):15–16.

170. Sandlin RE, Olsson RT. 2000. Subjective tinnitus: Its mechanisms and treatment. In: Valente M, Hosford-Dunn H, Roeser RJ, eds. *Audiology Treatment*. New York, NY: Thieme; 2000.

171. Newman, C W, Jacobson, GP. Application of self-report scales in balance function handicap assessment and management. *Sem Hear*. 1993;14(4):363–376.

172. Newman CW, Sandridge SA, Jacobson GP. Psychometric adequacy of Tinnitus Handicap Inventory for evaluating treatment outcome. J *Am Acad Audiol*. 1998;9:153–160.

173. Tyler RS. Neurophysiological models, psychological models, and treatment for tinnitus. In: Tyler RS, ed. *Tinnitus Treatment: Clinical Protocols*. New York, NY: Thieme; 2006:1–20.

174. Osaki Y, Nishimum HA, Takasawa M, et al. Neural mechanism of residual inhibition of tinnitus in cochlear implant users. *NeuroReport*. 2005;16(15):1625–1628.

175. Choy D. *Phase shift tinnitus reduction*. Presented at New York Academy of Medicine Symposium, New York; February 19, 2004.

176. Lipman RT, Lipman SP. Phase-shift treatment for predominant tone tinnitus. *Otolaryngol Head Neck Surg*. 2007;136: 763–768.

177. Noik E. *An effective solution for the treatment of tinnitus using phase-shift technology*. Presented at the European Federation of Audiology Societies, Gothenburg, Sweden; June 20, 2005.

178. Robb MJA. Tinnitus device directory, Part III. *Tinnitus Today*. 2006;31(1):14–16.

179. Robb MJA. Tinnitus device directory, Part IV. *Tinnitus Today*. 2006;31(2):9–12.

180. Goldstein B, Shulman A. Tinnitus evaluation. In: Shulman A, ed. *Tinnitus: Diagnosis/Treatment*. Philadelphia, Pa: Lea & Febiger; 1991.

181. Ayache D, Earally F, Elbaz, P. Characteristics and postoperative course of tinnitus in otosclerosis. *Otol Neurotol*. 2003; 24(1):48–51.

182. Gersdorff M, Nouwen J, Gilain C, et al. Tinnitus and otosclerosis. *Eur Arch Otorhinolaryngol*. 2000;257(6):314–316.

183. Sobrinho PG, Oliveira CA, Venosa AR. 2004. Long-term follow-up of tinnitus in patients with otosclerosis after stapes surgery. *Inter Tinnitus J*. 2004;10(2):197–201.

184. Jastreboff PJ. Phantom auditory perception (tinnitus): mechanisms of generation and perception. *Neurosci Res*. 1990;8: 221–254.

185. Jastreboff PJ, Hazell JWP. Treatment of tinnitus based on a neurophysiological model. In: Vernon J, ed. *Tinnitus: Treatment and Relief*. Boston, Mass: Allyn & Bacon; 1995.

186. Jastreboff PJ, Gray WL, Gold SL. Neurophysiological approach to tinnitus patients. *Am J Otol*. 1996;17:236–240.

187. Anderson G, Kaldo V. Cognitive-behavioral therapy with applied relaxation. In: Tyler RS, ed. *Tinnitus Treatment Clinical Protocols*. New York, NY: Thieme; 2006.

188. Beck J. *Cognitive Therapy: Basics and Beyond*. New York, NY: Guilford Press; 1995.

189. Henry JA, Wilson PH. The psychological management of tinnitus: comparison of a combined cognitive educational pro-

gram, education alone and a waiting-list control. *Int Tinnitus J.* 1996;1:9-20.

190. Newman CW, Sandridge SA. Incorporating group and individual sessions into a tinnitus management clinic. In: Tyler RS, ed. *Tinnitus Treatment: Clinical Protocols.* New York, NY: Thieme; 2005.

191. Henry JA, Loorin C, Montero M, et al. Tinnitus masking and tinnitus retraining combined. *J Rehab Res Develop.* 2007;44: 21-32.

192. Davis PB, Wilde RA, Steed L. Habituation-based rehabilitation technique using acoustic desensitization protocol. In: Patuzzi R, ed. *Proceedings of the Seventh International Tinnitus Seminar.* Perth: University of Western Australia; 2002:188-190.

193. Davis PB, Paki B, Hanley PJ. Neuromics tinnitus treatment: third clinical trial. *Ear Hear.* 2007;28:242-259.

194. Gagnier JJ, Boon H, Rochon P, et al. Reporting randomized controlled trials of herbal interventions: an elaborated consort statement. *Ann Intern Med.* 2006;144(5):364-367.

195. De Smet PAGM. Herbal remedies. *N Engl J Med.* 2002; 3347(25):2046-2056.

196. Rosenberg SI, Silverstein H, Rowan PT, et al. Effect of melatonin on tinnitus. *Laryngoscope.* 1998;103(3):30.

197. Megalu UC, Finnell JE, Piccirillo JF. The effects of melatonin on tinnitus and sleep. *Otolaryngol Head Neck Surg.* 2006; 134(2):210-213.

198. Drew S, Davies E. Effectiveness of Gingko biloba in treating tinnitus: double-blind, placebo controlled trial. *Birmingham Med J.* 2001;322:73.

199. Mayo Clinic. Ginkgo biloba. Retrieved September 2007 from http://www.mayoclinic.com/health/ginkgo-biloba/NS_patient-ginkgo

200. Johnson RM, Brummett R, Schleurning A. Use of Alphaprazolam for relief of tinnitus. A double-blind study. *Arch Otolaryngol Head Neck Surg.* 1993;119(8): 842-845.

201. http://www.stronghealth.com/services/tinnitus

202. Tyler RS, Coelho C, Noble W. Tinnitus: standard of care, personality differences, genetic factors. *J Otorhinolaryngol Relat Spec.* 2006;68:14-22.

203. Pulec JL, Hodell S, Anthony P. Tinnitus: diagnosis and treatment. *Ann Otol Rhinol Laryngol.* 1978;87:827-833.

204. Perry BP, Gantz BJ. Medical and surgical evaluation and management of tinnitus. In: Tyler R, ed. *Tinnitus Handbook*. San Diego, Calif: Singular; 2000:221–241.

205. Vernon JA, Schleuning AJ. Tinnitus: a new management. *Laryngol*. 1998;88(3):413–419.

# Section 1.4

# *Vestibular Disorders*

Auditory and vestibular functions are anatomic and physiologic neighbors. They share the same space (the otic capsule), bathe in similar lymph fluids, and convey their stimuli to the brain over adjacent portions of the same nerve (nVIII). But they serve different functions within the body.

The vestibular system (VS) consists of the semicircular canals, its nerve distribution, and portions of the brain, brainstem, and spinal cord. It provides stimuli that signal the body's positions in space and its acceleration/deceleration (proprioception). Its stimuli contribute to control of some muscles—like those of the eyes, head, and neck—and to maintaining balance. As with other parts of the central nervous system (CNS), auditory system and VS interact with each other.

## FREQUENCY OF OCCURRENCE

VS disorders in the population of United States are widespread: an estimated 20% of the general population is affected by a VS disorder, and an estimated half of the overall United States population is affected by a balance or VS disorder sometime during their lives.[1,2] Approximately 15 out of every 1,000 individuals consult their family physician each year with complaints that signal a VS disorder.[3]

Vestibular dysfunction is a prominent part of balance disorders, particularly in the elderly, and is a significant source of morbidity. It is estimated that half of persons over the age of 65 will develop positional vertigo, and half of the majority of falls they suffer probably will be due to VS disorders.[4]

A British study of hospital patients 18 to 64 years, in London, found dizziness, giddiness, vertigo, and unsteadiness in 480 of 2,064 cases (23%). That sizable rate of occurrence suggests that the incidence of VS disorder is probably much larger than estimated, although that finding should not be generalized, as it is based solely on a random sample of those who were hospitalized for unspecified conditions in one hospital.[5]

Estimates of the extent of persons with VS dysfunctions in the United States likely underestimate them. Counts depend on whether dysfunctions that are parts of other syndromes (e.g., Meniere's disease) are included in the estimates or are not also counted separately. Further statistical complications arise when the cause of a VS disorder cannot be established and when some of its symptoms are overlooked because they are mild and brief. In such cases, they are misreported or not reported at all to a physician or a survey interviewer, and therefore do not appear in accounts of their incidence or prevalence.[6]

Current statistics are collected and updated annually by the National Center for Health Statistics (NCHS), a U.S. government agency. The National Ambulatory Medical Care Survey and the National Center for Health Statistics are parts of the NCHS. Their publications are available on the Internet.[7]

## ETIOLOGY

VS disorders may be brought on by many causes; for example, strokes, tumors, degeneration of the cerebellum, toxins, head trauma, and as parts of diseases, such as, multiple sclerosis, otosclerosis, and Meniere's disease.[8]

Acute vestibular syndrome consists of vertigo, nausea, nystagmus, and postural instability. It typically results from injury to either peripheral or central vestibular structures, and it is usually attributed to viral vestibular neuritis. It may account for a sizable portion of emergency-room visits for severe vertigo, nausea, and vomiting.[9]

Vestibular neuronitis has been associated with sinusitis or an upper respiratory illness, but any inflammation of the vestibular nerve can cause it.[10] Maintenance of equilibrium, as another example, can be upset by inanition (starvation) and prolonged insomnia, as well as by the variety of causes mentioned above. Half of all falls suffered by the elderly are presumed to be the result of vestibular problems, thus associating disorders of the VS with aging of the VS.[11]

Benign paroxysmal positional vertigo (BPPV) is now believed to result from a lesion in the ampulla of a semicircular canal.[12] Reliable diagnostic signs have been codified, making it more likely that an underlying cause can be discovered.[13,14]

Structural genetic anomalies also result in VS disorder. Among these are aplasias and dysplasias associated with Mondini and Scheibe syndromes and cupulolithiasis and canalithiasis (see Section 1.2). Improved radiologic techniques have revealed these likely causes of some symptoms of VS disorder.

A somewhat mysterious condition bears the French name Mal de Debarquement (MDD—"disembarkment illness").[15] The patient who is affected by MDD has sensations of disequilibrium persisting for a lengthy period—months, even years—following an ocean voyage, airplane flight, or automobile journey. Such brief sensations are common among sailors and others who are subjected to prolonged rocking motions, but its chronic form is relatively rate. Treatment for MDD is empirical and often unavailing.

## DIAGNOSIS

Rehabilitation of VS disorders, as with the auditory disorders, begins with diagnosis.[16] Some diagnoses that have been used to characterize a broad group of conditions attributable to VS disorders are:

- Chronic vestibulopathy,
- Disequilibrium of aging,
- Postsurgical Imbalance,

- Labyrinthitis,
- Vestibular neuronitis,
- Connective tissue disorder,
- Bilateral vestibular weakness from ototoxicity, and
- Vertigo of unknown etiology.

Tests fail to make a diagnostic determination in from about one-third to one-half of patients with VS disorders.[17,18] A complete test battery might reduce this rate of indeterminacy in many instances, but obtaining such a detailed examination is not likely to occur if symptoms lack severity and are evanescent. Also, a thorough diagnosis sometimes can be uncomfortable for some patients and provoke symptoms in others, but obtaining an accurate picture of the underlying pathology is essential. Differential diagnosis of vestibular neuronitis, which is often initially mistaken for Meniere's disease, is made by absence of hearing loss and tinnitus. Vestibular neuronitis results from inflammation of the vestibulocochlear nerve. Labyrinthitis, which is caused by inflammation of the inner ear and has similar symptoms, usually is accompanied by hearing loss.[19] For that reason, a concurrent audiologic examination can help to delineate a symptom's etiologic basis. Clinicians faced with VS symptoms should consider evaluating the auditory system. Similarly, evaluating the VS can be rewarding in many cases of sensorineural hearing loss, especially in unusual cases in which the diagnosis may be in doubt.[20]

Clinicians need to be alert to the importance of evaluating the VS even in the absence of VS symptoms. That is certainly the case in patients with suspected acoustic neuroma, in which the balance evaluation may reveal diagnostic clues, although the patient may not express auditory complaints.

A complication for the diagnostician is that patients frequently present with more than one symptom; for example, vertigo and nystagmus often occur together. Hence, the importance of comprehensive examinations not only to be aware of the multiple symptoms, but also to lead to more accurate assessments of the patient's condition.[21]

When the patient complains of dizziness and imbalance, a critical investigatory tool is the neurotologic history. It focuses on how the symptoms are described, their temporal course, and any precursors that may have triggered them. Taken at bedside, its diagnostic impression can then be confirmed or denied by the laboratory tests, which are of limited value when isolated from the history.[22]

Clinicians have other diagnostic tools. Among these are electronystagmography and electro-oculography, computer dynamic posturography, the sensory organization test, and limits of stability testing.[23] New imaging techniques also have contributed to enhanced diagnoses, especially of CNS tumors.[24] Radiology will likely continue to improve on the presently advanced procedures and equipment.

## Dizziness and Vertigo

Diagnosis for patients presenting with dizziness and vertigo tends to be complicated and complex. Maintaining equilibrium requires obtaining and integrating information from visual, somatosensory, and vestibular systems. Dysfunction of any of these systems can cause the disequilibrium, but compensatory actions of the other two can obscure the location of the lesion. To improve diagnosis under such circumstances requires analyzing the inputs from each system—a procedure that can be taxing for both the patient and the clinician.[25]

## Differentiating Between Dizziness and Vertigo

Distinguishing between complaints of dizziness and vertigo assumes critical significance in planning treatment and subsequent rehabilitation.[26] The two terms are sometimes treated as synonymous, but maintaining the distinction between them is not only semantically proper, it can also facilitate management.[27]

Dizziness refers to a sensation of unsteadiness associated with movements within the head. It is a common, chronic, and often untreated symptom in adults. It typically does not arouse great anxiety in the patient, and it tends to be relatively common, especially among elderly people who move quickly from sitting or lying to an erect posture (positional or postural dizziness). The latter is largely due to vascular insufficiency within the VS. Other potential causes of dizziness are mild intoxication, emotional situations, vestibular neuritis, and head trauma. Some large acoustic neuromas also affect balance and may provoke dizziness, although it is not a frequent presenting symptom of early, small lesions of the vestibular portion of the eighth nerve (nVIII).[28]

Chronic dizziness offers further opportunities for differential diagnoses. It has been suggested that it be named chronic *subjective* dizziness.[29,30] Its most frequent causes are anxiety disorders, migraine, traumatic brain injury, and dysautonomia. Differentiating these etiologies can direct treatments for each cause—precursors to successful management.[31]

Vertigo, in contrast, arouses patients' extreme concern; its presence can be debilitating. Patients feel the surroundings are revolving around them (objective vertigo) or that they are rotating in space (subjective vertigo). It is frequently accompanied by nausea and vomiting and followed by fatigue and lassitude. When under a vertiginous attack, patients will refuse to move, even if they are lying in their own vomit, fearing that changing their position will exacerbate the symptom.

Vertigo has numerous causes. It is a component of diseases, like Meniere's, epilepsy, organic brain damage, cardiac, ocular, and gastric disorders, and systemic infections. When no specific cause can be identified, the condition is referred to as *essential vertigo*, in which case treatment may be empirical or trial-and-error; for example, antinausea medication that may provide symptomatic relief. Patients will usually insist on some form of relief, regardless of the rationale for it. Vertigo is a symptom that evokes strong responses from those affected by it.[32]

## Balance

A major function of the VS is maintaining balance. Disequilibrium is a serious consequence of vestibular damage, whether due to trauma, medication, or disease. Unsteadiness in dark-ness is typical of persons who are deaf and depend on visual stimuli to adjust their position and maintain their balance when in motion.[33]

## Nystagmus

Nystagmus (rapid, involuntary eye movements) by itself seldom brings patients to clinicians' attention because it rarely upsets patients, who usually do not see objects as moving despite the optical oscillations. The fact that perception remains essen-tially normal is probably due to cerebral adjustments in the interpretation of the fluctuating stimuli.[34]

By itself, nystagmus is not pathognomonic; however, it sig-nals underlying VS pathology and, when observed, should prompt vigorous investigation to identify the cause.[35] Also, distinguishing between oculomotor and amaurotic nystagmus (which occurs in cases of blindness or severely reduced visual ability) and between congenital and acquired nystagmus may be useful in directing treatment.[36]

## MANAGEMENT

Treatment of patients with VS disorders has advanced consid-erably in recent years. Formerly, they were either told to "do the best you can to live with your symptoms" or they were offered medicine and surgery. The former was frequently inad-equate, especially in severe cases, and the latter involved abla-tion that was irreversible, even if unhelpful.[37]

Confronted by these options, patients often sought multi-ple consultations from several clinicians. Today, however, they are likely to be given a fourth option: vestibular rehabilitation (VR).[38] These have several variations, but they place control over symptoms in the patients' hands.[39] Slow to be adopted, these exercises have now become a significant part of VR.[40]

Audiologists, physical therapists, and otologists may be involved in aspects of VR. It has become a full-time activity for many audiologists in private practice, though by no means all. They often treat benign positional paroxysmal vertigo (BPPV), as well as diagnosing other vestibular disorders. Although some authorities argue that the audiologist's and speech/language pathologist's scope of practice should be defined by communicative function, others assert that the anatomic origins of vestibular maladies place their assessment and rehabilitation within their purview.[41,42]

Once a patient is found to be vulnerable to VS disorders, examinations are recommended at least annually. These and more frequent visits seek to anticipate further damage and to evaluate treatments.[43] They provide opportunities to continue patients' education in techniques for ameliorating some aspects of VS disorders and avoiding others, and they can ensure that recommended exercises are being properly performed and faithfully carried out.[44] Providing patients with instructions and counseling them in order to alleviate emotional aspects of their symptoms can greatly assist patients to adjust to conditions for which no immediate therapies can eliminate their causes.

## Rehabilitation of Dizziness

Rehabilitation of dizziness frequently involves watchful waiting to determine if another attack occurs and, if not, instructing the patient how to escape similar incidents; for example, to avoid postural dizziness, the patient should move slowly from a recumbent to erect posture. Learning such a simple maneuver spares many elderly patients from injuries due to disastrous falls —a leading cause of injury and even death in older persons.[45]

Careful history taking will enable clinicians to identify other precursors and lead them to counsel their patients in techniques likely to avoid further incidents of dizziness or lightheadedness. These techniques include oculomotor, balance, and gait exercises.[46]

The Epley maneuver aims to correct benign paroxysmal postural vertigo (BPPV)—a condition that has been attributed to debris in the inner ear arising in the utricle (otoconia or "ear rocks"). In most instances, BPPV is incorrectly referred to as an instance of vertigo. The Epley maneuver moves the debris by head movements in four planes, each for about 30 seconds—a procedure is usually conducted in the practitioner's office. The Brandt-Daroff Exercises have basically the same rationale, but they are applied only when the Epley is unsuccessful. Requiring more time and being undertaken more vigorously, they can be done at home.[47]

## Rehabilitation of Vertigo

Rehabilitation of vertigo typically requires therapy for the underlying cause(s). Those associated with cardiovascular diseases respond well to exercises that come under the heading of Vestibular Rehabilitation Therapy, a group of noninvasive techniques that can be effective in treating vertigo.[48-51]

## Rehabilitation of Balance Disorders

Wavering gait, inability to maintain position in space, and other evidence of balance disorders may be alleviated by VR exercises. These may be needed following withdrawal from toxic reactions to drugs and other causes. Balance disorders sometimes arise following surgery and prolonged bed rest. In the latter instances, however, it is usually transient and requires no specific treatment beyond caution against falls.

## Rehabilitation of Nystagmus

As noted above, this condition has no single cause, nor is it usually amenable to therapy. In cases of congenital nystagmus, there is a possibility that surgery severing oculomotor muscles may eliminate it.[52]

Children whose nystagmus may interfere with their ability to read can be aided by the use of a card with a rectangular hole through which to observe the text. Other means that limit their viewing to one letter or line at a time can also be helpful.

Such tactics usually can be discarded as the child matures, as they tend to slow the reading process and make it more laborious.

## ADDITIONAL RESOURCES

Patients and their families may contact the Acoustic Neuroma Patient Archive for accounts of the experiences of persons with acoustic neuromas.[53] Those with vestibular disorders may wish to join the Vestibular Ear Disorder Association (Veda) to obtain current information and to make contacts with similarly afflicted individuals.[54] Another organization that serves like purposes is the American Hearing Organization that also serves persons with related vestibular problems as well as hearing disorders.[55] For recent updates, see the National Institute on Deafness and Other Communicative Disorders at http://www.nicd.gov .

## REFERENCES

1. University of Iowa Health Care. Comprehensive management of vestibular disorders. *Currents*: 2002;3(2). Retrieved Mar 2003 from http://www.uihealthcare.com/news/currents/vol3 issue2/03vertigo.html
2. Clinical Information: prevalence of balance and mobility disorders: vestibular disorders. Retrieved February 2007 from http://www.onbalance.com/clinical_info/prevalence/vestibular.aspx
3. Duke University Medical Center. Vestibular Rehabilitation Program. Retrieved Mar 2003 from http://www.dukehealth.org/ptot/vestibular_ rehab.asp
4. Ator GA. University of Kansas Department of Otolaryngology Division of Otology Vertigo: evaluation and treatment in the elderly. Retrieved March 2003 from http://www2.kumc.edu/otolaryngology/otology/VertEldTalk.htm
5. Yardley L, Owen N, Nazareth I. Prevalence and presentation of dizziness in a general practice community sample of working age people. *Br J Gen Pract*. 1998;48(429):1131–1135.
6. Kerber KA, Brown DL, Lisabeth LD, et al. Stroke among patients with dizziness, vertigo and imbalance in the emer-

gency department. A population-based study. *Stroke*. 2006;37: 2484-2487.

7. Health Statistics. Retrieved April 2007 from http://www.cdc. gov/nchs

8. Herdman SJ. *Vestibular Rehabilitation*. 3rd ed. Philadelphia, Pa: FA Davis; 2007.

9. Hotson JR, Baloh RW. Acute vestibular syndrome. *N Engl J Med*. 1998;339:680-685.

10. Gacek RR, Gacek MR. Vestibular neuronitis: a viral neuropathy. *Adv Otorhinolaryngol*. 2002;60:54-66.

11. Rubenstein LZ. Falls in older people: epidemiology, risk factors and strategies for prevention. *Age Ageing*. 2006;35(suppl 2): 37-41.

12. Epley J. BPPV diagnosis and management. *Vestib Update: Micromed Technol* 1992;8:1-4.

13. Black FO, Nasher LM. Postural disturbances in patients with benign paroxysmal positional nystagmus. *Ann Otol Rhinol Laryngol*. 1984;93:595-599.

14. Fife TD. Recognition and management of horizontal canal benign positional vertigo. *Am J Otol*. 1998;19(3):345-351.

15. Gordeon CR, Spitzer O, Doweck I, et al. Clinical features of mal de debarquement: adaptation and habituation to sea conditions. *J Vestib Res*. 1995;5(5):363-369.

16. Herdman SJ, ed. *Vestibular Rehabilitation*. 2nd ed. Philadelphia, Pa: FA Davis; 2000.

17. Hain TC. 1995. Treatment of vertigo. *Neurologist*. 1:125-133.

18. Weiss AH, Phillips JO. Congenital and compensated vestibular dysfunction in childhood: an overlooked entity. *J Child Neurol*. 2006;21:572-579.

19. Gacek RR, Gacek MR. Some characteristics of vertigo in vestibular neuronitis. *Vestib Otorinolaringol*. 2004;6:18-21.

20. Boenki J, Rambold H, Stritzke G, et al. Vestibular dysfunction in acute unilateral hearing loss. *Ann NY Acad Sci*. 2003;1004: 482-484.

21. Shephard NT. Dizziness and balance disorders: the role of history and laboratory studies in diagnosis and management. *ASHA Leader*. 2007;12(7):6-7,16-17.

22. Delaney KA. Bedside diagnosis of vertigo: value of the history and neurological examination. *Acad Emerg Med*. 2003;10: 1388-1395.

23. Bauer CA, Girardi M. Vestibular rehabilitation. Retrieved 2/26/06 from http://www.emedicine.com/ent/topic666.htm

24. Baehring JM, Piepmeier JM. *Brain Tumors: Practical Guide to Diagnosis and Treatment*. New York, NY: Informa; 2007.

25. Dieterich M. Dizziness. *Neurologist*. 2004;10(3):154–164.

26. Dix M. Rehabilitation of vertigo. In: Dix MR, Hood JD, eds. *Vertigo*. New York, NY: John Wiley & Sons; 1984.

27. Shephard NT. Differentiation of Meniere's disease and migraine-associated dizziness. *J Am Acad Audiol*. 2006;17:69–80.

28. Jacobson GP, Newman CW. The development of the dizziness handicap inventory. *Arch Otolaryngol Head Neck Surg*. 1990; 116:424–427.

29. Staab JP, Ruckenstein MJ, Amsterdam JD. A prospective trial of sertaline for chronic subjective dizziness. *Laryngoscope*. 2004;114:1637–1641.

30. Staab JP, Ruckenstein MJ. Chronic dizziness and anxiety course of illness affects treatment outcome. *Arch Otolaryngol Head Neck Surg*. 2005;131:675–679.

31. Staab JP. Expanding the differential diagnosis of chronic dizziness. *Arch Otolaryngol Head Neck Surg*. 2007;133:170–176.

32. Hain TC. Treatment of vertigo. *Neurologist*. 1995;1:125–133.

33. Shepard NT, Telian SA. *Practical Management of the Balance Disorder*. San Diego, Calif: Singular; 1995.

34. Abadi RV. Mechanisms underlying nystagmus. *J Roy Soc Med*. 2002;96:231–234.

35. Serra A, Leigh RJ. Diagnostic value of nystagmus: spontaneous and induced ocular oscillations. *J Neurol Neurosurg Psychiatr*. 2002:73:615–618.

36. Stuhl JS, Auerbach-Heller L, Leigh J. Acquired nystagmus. *Arch Ophthalmol*. 2000;118:544–549.

37. Curthoys IS, Halmagyi GM. How does the brain compensate for vestibular lesions? In: Baloh RW, Halmagyi GM, eds. *Disorders of the Vestibular System*. New York, NY: Oxford University Press; 1996:145–154.

38. Desmond AL. Vestibular rehabilitation. In Roeser RJ, Valente M, Hosford-Dunn H. *Audiology Treatment*. New York, NY: Thieme; 2000.

39. McCabe BF. Labyrinthine exercises in the treatment of diseases characterized by vertigo. Their physiologic basis and methodology. *Laryngoscope*. 1970;80:1429–1433.

40. Norre ME, Beckers A. Comparative study of two types of exercise treatment for paroxysmal positioning vertigo. *Ann Otol, Rhinol Laryngol.* 1988;42:287–289.

41. Shepard NT, Garrus NP, Hecker EB, et al. Role of audiologists in vestibular and balance rehabilitation: American Speech-Language-Hearing Association: position statement, guidelines, and technical report. *Asha.* 1999;41(suppl 19):13–22.

42. Martin FN, Clark JG. *Introduction to Audiology.* 9th ed. Boston, Mass: Pearson Education; 2006.

43. Shumway-Cook A, Gruber W, Baldwin MS, et al. The effect of multidimensional exercises on balance, mobility, and fall risk in community-dwelling older adults. *Phys Ther.* 1997;77:46–57.

44. Carter S, Laird C. Assessment and care of ENT problems. *Emerg Med J.* 2005;22:128–129.

45. Drachman DA, Hart CW. An approach to the dizzy patient. *Neurology.* 1972;22:323–333.

46. Badke MB, Miedaner JA, Shea TA, et al. Effects of vestibular and balance rehabilitation on sensory organization and dizziness handicap. *Ann Otol Rhinol Laryngol.* 2005;114: 48–54.

47. Herdman SJ, ed. *Vestibular Rehabilitation.* 3rd ed. Philadelphia, Pa: FA Davis; 2007.

48. Brockwell CW. *ENG Workbook.* Baltimore, Md: University Park Press; 1983.

49. Brockwell CW, Bojrab DI. Background and technique of rotational testing. In: Jacobson GP, Newman CP, Kartush JM, eds. *Handbook of Balance Function Testing.* St. Louis, Mo: Mosby; 1993.

50. McCabe BF. Labyrinthine exercises in the treatment of diseases characterized by vertigo. Their physiologic basis and methodology. *Laryngoscope.* 1970;80:1429–1433.

51. Wazen JJ, Mitchell D. *Dizzy.* New York, NY: Simon & Schuster; 2004.

52. Dell'Osso LF, Hertle RW, Williams RW, et al. A new surgery for congenital nystagmus: effects of tenotomy on an achiasmatic canine and the role of extraocular proprioception. *J AAPOS.* 1999;3:166–182.

53. Acoustic Neuroma Patient Archive. Retrieved 2/2007 from http://www.anarchive.org/vestibular_rehab

54. Veda. Retrieved 8/2007 from http://www.vestibular.org

55. American Hearing Organization. Retrieved 8/2007 from http://www.american-hearing.org

# SECTION 2

# Management Options

The following subsections address broadly the subject of treatment of hearing losses. These are divided into three subsections: 2.1, Amplification; 2.2, Cochlear Implants; and 2.3, Compensation Strategies.

## SECTION 2.1: AMPLIFICATION

The most common therapeutic response to sensorineural hearing loss is amplification—providing increased sound pressure and intelligibility to the affected ear or ears. The general approach in Section 2.1 applies to most disorders and supplements any discussions of amplification that apply only to a specific disorder.

## SECTION 2.2: COCHLEAR IMPLANTS

In recent years, another option has appeared, the cochlear implant (CI). Section 2.2 presents aspects of this device, which stimulates the auditory nerve with electrical impulses corresponding to environmental sounds, including speech, that surround the patient with hearing loss.

Most of patients with CI learn to interpret the electrical impulses as if they were hearing the sounds that generated them. Recently, new adaptations of CI have been introduced to deal with disabilities that require special versions. These are needed to apply to conditions like von Recklinghausen disease and some of the aplasias.

## SECTION 2.3: STRATEGIES TO COMPENSATE FOR HEARING LOSS

In Section 2.3, a variety of techniques available to the clinician are presented. Although amplification and CI provide direct means of overcoming the reduced ability of the ear or ears to process sounds meaningfully, there are additional strategies and tactics that can assist patients with hearing losses to conduct activities of daily living in more effective ways. They supplement the instrumental approaches. The discussion of the compensatory activities is intended to add to the specifics that are especially relevant to each of the conditions presented in Sections 1.1 and 1.2. Although all patients should receive counseling to help them adjust to their lost or reduced ability to hear, both emotionally and intellectually, they can also develop or improve speechreading skills, learn to use alternative forms of communication, acquire education about ways to conserve their speech and residual hearing, and more.

## THE FUTURE

Unlike Alexander the Great, hearing rehabilitators need not cry, "There are no worlds left to conquer!" Ample challenges remain.

### Ultrasonic Hearing Aids

Can the frequencies over 20,000 Hz be used to stimulate the eighth nerve? Such high-frequency vibrations applied directly to the head might produce a detectable response that, like the electrical impulses generated by cochlear implants, can be used as a hearing analog.[1] The idea is currently being researched.[2]

## Mechanical Cochlea

Another possible advance in providing amplification is the mechanical cochlea designed to function like its human counterpart. When available, its advantages over other artificial cochleas will likely be that it (a) can be mass produced, (b) is only 3 cm long, and (c) has no moving parts.[3]

## Counseling and Education

Counseling and education have critical roles to play in hearing rehabilitation. We urge that treatment go beyond dispensing aids and medications. Nor should hearing rehabilitation end with a prescription or a fitting. Patient follow-up to ensure the efficacy of treatment should be included in the rehabilitation design.

## REFERENCES

1. Cere Biotechnology. Retrieved October 2007 from http://www.vabiotech.com/parknews/news_release/release_2006_01_23.html
2. Mosheim J. Ultrasonic hearing: expanding human limitations. *Advance for Speech-Language Pathologists and Audiologists.* 2006;16(6):6–8, 20.
3. University of Michigan develops mechanical cochlea. Retrieved October 2007 from http://www.sciencedaily.com/releases/2005/02/050205104015.htm

# Section 2.1

# *Amplification*

Amplification is a prime component of the rehabilitation program, predominantly serving persons with sensorineural hearing losses associated with a variety of distortions; for example, loudness recruitment, narrowed range of uncomfortable loudness, and deterioration in the ability to discriminate speech, especially in noisy backgrounds.[1] Conductive hearing losses are now largely alleviated by surgery.

The extensive changes in hearing aids make the choice of instrument important, but even the best available hearing aids do not completely overcome sensorineural hearing losses. More critical than the instrument is a knowledgeable clinician who can lead the patient to accept the need for assistance and can recommend appropriate aid. That is why ongoing counseling, educational programs, and reprogramming must be added to the increasingly complex hardware and software that are essential to successful rehabilitation.[2]

## THE PREFITTING EXAMINATION

In addition to comprehensive audiologic diagnosis, the initial hearing-aid evaluation should also assess the patient's motivation and determine usual listening conditions—procedures that require time and, perhaps, more than one visit.[3] Hearing inventories and questionnaires completed by patients and their significant others can be helpful in collecting and organizing these and related data.[4,5]

Delivering the results of the comprehensive examination should be done with care. For example, most patients can more easily grasp test results expressed in percentages than in decibels or other unfamiliar metrics. Brochures written in a friendly manner can also be helpful.[6]

When the following "red flags" are observed in the audiologic examination, dispensing should be deferred until additional diagnostic procedures have been performed:

■ Asymmetric pure-tone loss in which one ear is poorer by as little as 10 to 15 dB, even when the sensorineural function of the poorer ear falls within normal limits;

■ Significant difference between ears in word-recognition (discrimination) scores;

■ Unilateral or asymmetric findings on a stapedial-reflex measure or stapedial-reflex decay;

■ Tinnitus that is unilateral, asymmetric or changing in quality in persons with long-standing hearing loss.

These symptoms may arise from retrocochlear pathology that requires medical/surgical intervention.

Children who appear not to be functioning well with their hearing aids should receive a complete audiologic examination, including tympanometry, and referred to a pediatric otologist for treatment. The existence of an additional effusion-related conductive component may be signaled by feedback from the child's hearing aid that was previously not present.

Of cardinal importance is beginning treatment promptly. Evidence has shown that congenitally hard-of-hearing and deaf infants who receive appropriate rehabilitation measures before 6 months of age maintain language development commensurate with their cognitive abilities at least through age 5 years.[7]

When is amplification indicated? The Pediatric Working Group recommended amplification for children with pure-tone thresholds equal to or greater than 25 dB HL.[8] Children with unilateral high-frequency hearing loss above 2000 to 3000 Hz and those with milder hearing loss should be evaluated on a case-by-case basis with consideration of such factors as cognitive function, existence of other disabilities, and how well the child is doing at home or in a classroom environment.[9]

## Basic Components of Hearing Aids[10]

Hearing aids are a collection of components that justify calling the resulting instrument an amplification system.[11] Each commercial hearing aid will have components that are unique to its brand, although all hearing aids will have the following classic components.[12]

### *Microphone*

Sound waves enter the hearing aid through the microphone, which converts the acoustical into an electronic signal. This component can limit the amount of amplified low-frequency energy. Directional microphones favor signals originating from in front of the hearing aid with as much as a 20 dB gain over those originating behind it, which can improve the signal-to-noise ratio by as much as 6 dB, and which can be incorporated in all but the smallest instruments.[13,14]

### *Amplifier*

The amplifier increases the strength of the electrical signal. Its placement within the structure of the instrument and its capacity depend on the manufacturer's design.[15]

### *Receiver*

The receiver is a miniature loudspeaker that converts the amplified signal back into sound waves. The amplified sound directed from the receiver into the user's external auditory canal may affect the high-frequency response.

### *Battery*

The electrical energy that powers the hearing aid and allows the amplification process to occur is a battery.

### *Controls and Features*

Hearing aids have controls that increase their adaptability to individual preferences and optimal hearing requirements. These include:

- a telecoil, which is a special circuit enabling the aid to be used with a telephone, but that cannot be incorporated completely in in-the-canal hearing aids, because of its small size;
- a volume control that can be programmed to adjust for loudness variations, found in some, though not all, digital hearing aids;
- data logging, which has been built into some digital hearing aids, to determine the amount of time spent in different listening situations.

The American National Standards Institute publishes specifications for additional characteristics of importance to patients; for example, high-frequency average, full-on gain, harmonic distortion, and compression.[16]

### Analog Versus Digital Instruments

Digital hearing aids have replaced the analog.[17] Their principal advantages are fitting flexibility—the ability to adjust the aid to listening conditions—and algorithms for feedback cancellation.

The essence of their advantage is Digital Signal Processing (DSP) that provides as many as 32 channels of signal processing. Furthermore, digital over analog hearing aids offer quieter complex circuitry with lesser battery drain. DSP encourages fine tuning that can be done accurately, after patients report to the clinician about their hearing experiences in various listening conditions (see "The Postfitting Consult" below). Directional microphones also improve the digital hearing aid's ability to effectively reproduce speech in noise. Another feature is limitation of the feedback problem.[18]

Multichannel compression allows for greater control of the frequency response.[19] Compression is the concentration of the amplification into the patient's dynamic range of hearing; the input signal is compressed at a preset level in a nonlinear fashion to produce a reduced range of output. It is a type of automatic gain control that promotes more effective noise suppression and feedback management. Most digital hearing aids have this feature.

## Instrument Sizes, Types, and Placements

Hearing aids come in several configurations and incorporate different features, as noted above. The choice of hearing-aid style depends on the nature of the hearing loss and the patient's personal preferences. These have ranged from a hand cupped behind the ear, to ear trumpets, to today's highly sophisticated electronic instruments.

### *Implantable Hearing Aids*

In recent years, both partially and fully implantable hearing aids have been developed. They bypass the external auditory canal and directly vibrate the ossicular chain.[20]

One such device is designed for adults with congenital auricular atresia. It appears to have succeeded in those with an air-bone gap of 50 to 60 dB.[21] In a study of 20 persons, researchers found that the Otologic's MET Fully-Implantable Ossicular Stimulator provides an alternative to currently available hearing aids for persons with moderate-to-severe sensorineural hearing losses.[22]

## Body-Worn and Eyeglass Hearing Aids

The body-worn hearing aid can generate enough acoustic gain for those with severe-to-profound hearing losses. Eyeglass hearing aids embed the amplifier and receiver in the temporal portions of the eyeglass frame. Plastic tubing then conveys the input to the ear. Body-worn and eyeglass aids have now largely been replaced by smaller hearing aids having equal or greater power than body-worn aids and that are less obtrusive than eyeglass aids.

## Behind-the-Ear (BTE) and In-the-Ear (ITE) Hearing Aids

BTE aids contain the microphone, amplifier, and battery in one unit small and light enough to be worn. The receiver sends the amplified sound into a plastic tube attached to a custom-fitted earmold.

ITE aids have circuitry built into the earmold, so the entire instrument fits into the external ear. Although originally limited to persons with mild hearing losses, ITE's designs have made them feasible for those with moderate-to-moderately severe hearing losses. A variation of the ITE aid fits completely in the canal (CIC), a design that takes full advantage of the natural acoustic properties of the pinna and is appropriate for persons with hearing loss in the mild-to-moderate range. However, CIC aids are too small to accommodate telecoils.

For children with significant hearing losses who need access to FM systems in the classroom, BTE aids with telecoils continue to be the fitting of choice. Some adults with normal to near-normal hearing in the low frequencies and moderate hearing losses in the high frequencies prefer open-canal fitting. The tip from a very small BTE aid is inserted into the ear canal and connected to the earmold, which is a shell that does not block the ear canal, virtually eliminating the occlusion effect and accentuating venting.[23]

## FITTING CHILDREN

The selection and fitting of hearing aids is the primary rehabilitative tool for the overwhelming majority of children with varying degrees of sensorineural hearing loss. Intervention should be started by 6 months of age for those with hearing loss identified and evaluated at birth or during the neonatal period.

Audiologic intervention up to 6 months of age will rely primarily on ABR with threshold searching for pure-tone thresholds at key frequencies needed to determine the hearing-aid responses and otoacoustic emissions (OAE). As ABR and OAE do not require volitional responses from the infant being evaluated, the information provided by these procedures suffices for prescription of amplification, which should not be delayed until audiometric are available. (See "Infant Screening" in Section 1 Introduction.)

The Pediatric Working Group recommends amplification for children with pure-tone thresholds equal to or greater than 25 dB HL. Children with unilateral high-frequency hearing loss above 2 to 3000 Hz and those with milder hearing loss should be evaluated on a case-by-case basis with consideration of such factors as cognitive function, existence of other disabilities, and how well the child is doing at home or in a classroom environment.

Basic principles guiding the fitting of hearing aids on infants and young children less than 6 months of age through early childhood are:

- Fit bilaterally even when there is an asymmetric loss, with few exceptions.[24]
- Because the pinna and external ear canal grow, often rapidly, the style of choice is a behind-the-ear, not an in-the-ear, hearing aid. As the anatomy changes, only a change in earmold will be necessary.
- Hearing aids should be programmable and fully digital. Because the audiometric configuration may not be

known at the beginning of the fitting process, the flexibility of these aids is an advantage during periods of increased hearing loss from bouts of otitis media. The hearing loss may fluctuate, and flexible reprogramming makes possible adjustments to changes in frequency response and gain.[25]

The Desired Sensation Level formula (DSL) targets sensation levels for amplified speech; that is, the number of decibels above threshold at which speech intelligibility can be maximized yet remain comfortable. This value is defined in real-ear sound-pressure levels to control for individual ear-canal acoustics and earmold resonances. The resulting difference between real-ear threshold and real-ear-target-aided level is the DSL for amplified speech.[26,27]

## AMPLIFICATION FOR PATIENTS WITH UNILATERAL LOSSES

The clinician has several options for treating patients with unilateral or one-sided hearing loss.[28] If there is adequate residual hearing in the affected ear, an ITE or BTE hearing aid for that ear may be prescribed. If the affected ear lacks sufficient residual hearing, a contralateral routing of offside signals aid (CROS) or a bone-anchored cochlear stimulator (BAHA) surgically implanted in the affected ear may be prescribed.[29] One study found greater patient satisfaction and improved communication with BAHA over CROS aids.[30]

## FITTING OLDER PATIENTS

Following the arrival of hearing aids ordered for the older patient, the first visit should deal with basic instruction on care and maintenance of the instrument. The fit of the aid or earmold is carefully checked, as undue pressure on the skin of the auditory canal may lead to abandonment of the entire device, not uncommon, especially among males who resent and reject the process and may be going along with it to "please" their spouses on get them "off their necks."

The hearing aids are programmed with a computer for real-word listening situations. Instruments with multiple memory switches are extremely important, as they allow different frequency responses for different communication situations; for example, in quiet, a noisy auditorium, the telephone. Patients should be instructed to keep diaries of their experiences with each program to be reviewed with the patient at the next visit, at which time fine tuning of each program based on patients' experiences are incorporated into the hearing aid's digitalized circuitry. During the trial period, sessions should be scheduled frequently. Subsequent to the trial period, regularly scheduled sessions devoted to further reprogramming and audiologic rehabilitation should be scheduled. The infinitely readjustable changes that are possible with fully digitalized amplification are both an advantage and a potential problem. As even the best quality amplification never equals unaided, normal hearing or the recollection of how they once heard, patients may search for a level of performance that is unachievable. Even in this era, realistic expectations must be established; otherwise patients will not make a positive adjustment to their hearing losses. The dispenser must direct the search for an attainable audiologic dream.

## Acclimatization

Auditory acclimatization is an improvement in auditory function as a result of increased loudness being presented to the listener.[31] A comparison of wide dynamic range, multichannel compression with linear amplification found that acclimatization appears to depend on the type of amplification and previous experience with amplification.[32]

Improvement in the accuracy of speech recognition takes from 4 to 6 weeks, although the acclimatization process takes longer for many seniors, requiring follow-up visits to assist them in adapting to real-world listening situations.[33] The Food and Drug Administration recommends the 4-to-6-week acclimatization period after obtaining amplification for confirming the effectiveness of hearing aids.[34]

## ASSISTIVE LISTENING DEVICES

Assistive listening devices (ALD) are amplification systems that can assist or replace hearing aids in conditions of loud background noise, overlapping conversations, speech degradation from excessive room reverberations, and long distances from sound sources, especially in large assembly areas.[35] ALD with FM can also provide improvement in understanding speech in difficult listening environments with unilateral hearing loss.[36]

The Americans with Disabilities Act recognizes the handicapping nature of these conditions for persons with impaired hearing and requires public facilities to provide ALDs.[37] However, many clinicians do not offer them, and persons who could profit from ALD often do not appear to be aware of their potential benefits.[38] To encourage further use of ALD, the government sponsors four regional centers of information and assistance, referred to as Pep-Net.[39]

Each type of ALD has advantages and disadvantages, but all improve the signal-to-noise ratio.

### Hard-Wire Versus Wireless ALD

Hardwire ALDs use direct electrical connection to transmit auditory signals. Induction loop systems connect the speaker's microphone to an amplifier connected to a magnetic core. The signal then can be received by the telecoil in a hearing aid.

Wireless units transmit via radio frequencies, light waves (infrared systems), or via magnetic induction. FM systems are often portable and battery-operated. They are found predominantly in classes for deaf and hard-of-hearing students. The teacher or speaker wears a microphone connected to a body-worn transmitter that sends the voice to one or more receivers or hearing aids in the immediate vicinity. Special FM systems can be used with cochlear-implant users and in conjunction with behind-the-ear hearing aids. Monitoring by audiologists is necessary to avoid damage to the listeners' ears by intense transmission of sound.[40]

Infrared systems (IRS) use a wireless microphone that signals a transmitter that sends an invisible infrared light to receivers worn by listeners that convert the light signal to sound. They are largely found in theaters, houses of worship, and large auditoriums.[41]

## Sound-Field Amplification

Sound-field amplification systems do not require users to wear receivers. The speaker has a microphone that connects to a loudspeaker mounted on the ceiling or wall. All listeners—whether with normal or subnormal hearing—receive the speech without any stigma that may be attached to wearing a special device.[42] The extent to which such a system provides improved hearing depends, in large part, on the hearing abilities of the audience.

## TACTILE AIDS

Tactile aids respond to sounds by converting them to vibrations (vibrotactile aids) or electrical impulses (electrotactile aids), which are transmitted to the skin.[43] They require considerable instruction and practice to obtain their full benefits.[44]

They may be prescribed in place of cochlear implants or combined with them.[45] A case report of combined use of a hearing aid and a tactile aid found the combination improved lip reading and recognition of environmental sounds.[46] However, a larger study combining tactile aids and CIs reported outcomes that were not superior to CIs alone.[47]

## THE POSTFITTING CONSULTS

Follow-up meetings with patients to discuss problems with their aids and to adjust their aids' programming reduce dissatisfaction and forestall future problems.[48] More studies of disappointed hearing-aid consumers are needed to understand what factors account for their dissatisfaction. See "Strategies to Compensate for Hearing Loss" in Section 2.3 for the postfitting visits that should be scheduled parts of hearing rehabilitation.

## REFERENCES

1. Mueller HG, Johnson EE, Carter AS. Hearing aids and assistive devices. In: Schow RL, Nerbonne MA, eds. *Introduction to Audiologic Rehabilitation*. 5th ed. Boston, Mass: Allyn & Bacon; 2007.

2. Valente M, Valente LM, Hullar T. Problems and solutions for fitting amplification to patients with Meniere's disease. *J Am Acad Audiol*. 2006;17:6–15.

3. Valente M, Valente M. Hearing aid fitting and verification procedures for adults. In: Katz J, ed. *Handbook of Clinical Audiology*. 5th ed. Baltimore, Md: Lippincott Williams & Wilkins; 2002.

4. Ventry I, Weinstein B. The Hearing Handicap Inventory for the Elderly: a new tool. *Ear Hear*. 1982;83:128–134.

5. Saunders GH, Cienkowski KM, Forsline A, et al. Normative data for the Attitudes Towards Loss of Hearing Questionnaire. *J Am Acad Audiol*. 2005;16:637–652.

6. Martin FN, Clark JG. Amplification/sensory systems. In: Martin FA, Clark JG, eds. *Introduction to Audiology*, 9th ed. Boston, Mass: Allyn & Bacon; 2006.

7. Yoshinaga-Itano C, Sidey A, Coulter D, et al. Language of early and later identified children with hearing loss. *Pediatrics*. 1998;102:1161–1171.

8. Pediatric Working Group of the Conference on Amplification for Children with Auditory Deficits. Amplification for infants and children with hearing loss. *Am J Audiol*. 1996;5(1):53–68.

9. Killion MC. Talking hair cells: what they have to say about hearing aids. In: Berlin CL, ed. *Hair Cells and Hearing Aids*. San Diego, Calif: Singular; 1996.

10. Dillon H. *Hearing Aids*. New York, NY: Thieme; 2001.

11. Levitt H. A historical perspective on digital hearing aids: how digital technology has changed modern hearing aids. *Trends Amplification*. 2007;11(1):7-24.

12. Kuk F, Ludrigsen C. Changing with the times: choice of stimuli for hearing-aid verification, pure-tones, speech or composite signals? Here's what to use and why. *Hear Rev*. 2003;10(9):24-28, 56-57.

13. Ricketts TA. Directional hearing aids. *J Rehab Res Develop*. 2005;42(4, suppl 2):133-144.

14. Saunders GH, Fausti SA. Advanced hearing aid features: directional microphones and telecoils. *Sem Hear*. 2005;26(2): 57-124.

15. Mispagel KM, Valente M. Effect of multi-channel digital signal processing on loudness comfort, sentence recognition, and sound quality. *J Am Acad Audiol*. 2006;17(10):681-707.

16. American National Standards Institute. *Specification of Hearing Aid Characteristics*. (ANSI S3.22-2003). New York, NY: Acoustical Society of America; 2003.

17. Kim HH, Barry KD. Hearing aids: a review of what's new. *Otolaryngol Head Neck Surg*. 2006;134:1043-1050.

18. Parsa V. Acoustic feedback and its reduction through digital signal processing *Hear J*. 2006;59:11:16-23.

19. Agnew J. Hearing aid adjustments through potentiometer and switch options. In: Valente M, ed. *Hearing Aid Options and Limitations*. 2nd ed. New York, NY: Thieme; 2002:162-164.

20. Snik FM, Cremers WRJ. First audiometric results with the Vibrant Soundbridge, a semi-implantable hearing device for sensorineural hearing loss. *Audiology*. 1999;6:335-338.

21. Siegert R, Mattheis S, Kasic J. Fully implantable hearing aids in patients with congenital auricular atresia. *Laryngoscope*. 2007;117(2):336-340.

22. Jenkins HA, Atkins JS, Horlbeck D, et al. U.S. Phase I preliminary results of the Otologics MET Fully-Implantable ossicular stimulator. *Otolarygol Head Neck Surg*. 2007;137:206-212.

23. Mueller HG. Open is in. *Hear J*. 2006;259:11-14.

24. Simon HJ. Bilateral amplification and sound localizaton: then and now. *J Rehab Res Develop*. 2005;42(4, suppl 2):117-132.

25. Stach BA. *Clinical Audiology: An Introduction*. San Diego, Calif: Singular; 1998.

26. Seewald RC. The Desired Sensation Level method for hearing aid fitting in infants and children. *Phonak Focus*. 1996;20: 4-18.

27. Seewald RC, Moodie KS, Sinclair ST, et al. Predictive validity of a procedure for pediatric hearing instrument fitting. *Am J Audiol*. 2000;8(2):143-152.

28. Wazen JJ, Ghossaini SN. The diagnostic and treatment dilemma of sudden sensorineural hearing loss. *Hear Rev*. 2003;10(15):38-41.

29. Wazen JJ, Spitzer JB, Ghossaini SN, et al. Transcranial contralateral cochlear stimulation in unilateral deafness. *Otolaryngol Head Neck Surg*. 2003;129(3):248-254.

30. Miller MH, Schein JD. The forgotten ear. *Hear Hlth*. 1999; 15(4):18-20, 46.

31. Arlinger S, Gatehouse S, Bentler RA, et al. Report of the Eriksholm Workshop on auditory deprivations and acclimatization. *Ear Hear*. 1996;17(suppl 3):87S-90S.

32. Yund EW, Roup CM, Simon HJ, et al. Acclimatization in wide dynamic range multichannel compression and linear hearing aids. *J Rehab Res Develop*. 2006;43(4):517-536.

33. Surr RK, Cord MT, Walden BE. Long-term versus short-term hearing aid benefit. *J Am Acad Audiol*. 1998;9:165-171.

34. Food and Drug Administration. *Guidance for hearing aid manufacturers for substantiation claims*. Rockville, Md: Author; 1994.

35. Crandall CC, Smaldino J. Room acoustics and auditory rehabilitation technology. In: Katz J, ed. *Handbook of Clinical Audiology*. 5th ed. Baltimore, Md: Lippincott Williams & Wilkins; 2002.

36. Mahon W. Assistive devices and systems: the market lists. *Hear J*. 1985;38:7-13.

37. Americans with Disabilities Act. *Federal Register* 28 CFR Part 36. Washington DC: United States Government Printing Office;1991.

38. Jerger J. The development of assistive listening devices. *Aud Soc New Zealand Newsletter*. 1993;17:2.

39. PEPNet. Retrieved September 2007 from netac@rit.edu

40. American Speech/Language Hearing Association. Guidelines for acoustics in educational environments. *Asha*. 1995; 37(suppl 14D):15-19.

41. Malinoff R, Kisiel D, Kisiel S, Duggert P. The dispensing of hearing instruments: a study on industry structures and trends. *Hear Inst*. 1990;41:12-14.

42. Dibonis DA, Donohue CL. 2004. *Survey of Audiology*. Boston, Mass: Allyn & Bacon; 2004.

43. Committee on Hearing, Bioacoustics, and Biomechanics Working Group on Communication Aids for the Hearing Impaired (CHABA). Speech-perception aids for hearing-impaired people: current status and needed research. *J Acoust Soc Am*. 1191;90:637-685.

44. Gelfand SA. *Essentials of Audiology*. 2nd ed. New York, NY: Thieme; 2001.

45. Pickett J, MacFarland W. Auditory implants and tactile aids for the profoundly deaf. *J Speech Hear Res*. 1985;8:134-150.

46. Reed CM, Delhorne LA. A study of the combined use of a hearing aid and tactual aid in an adults with profound hearing loss. *Volta Rev*. 2006;106:171-193.

47. Geers A, Moog J. Effectiveness of CI and tactile aids for deaf children: the sensory aids study at the Central Institute for the Deaf. *Volta Rev*. 1994;96:5.

48. Saunders GH, Chisolm TH, Abram HB. Measuring hearing aid outcomes—not as easy as it seems. *J Rehab Res Develop*. 2005;42(4, suppl 2):157-168.

# Section 2.2

# *Cochlear Implants*

For patients with severe to profound hearing losses who do not gain sufficient benefit from conventional amplification, the cochlear implant (CI) opens another rehabilitation option.

## BRIEF HISTORY OF CI

Direct electrical stimulation of the auditory portion of nVIII to simulate hearing was first recorded by two French otologists, in 1957.[1] In 1965, the first permanent implant was reported in the United States.[2] The House-Urban single-electrode device followed it.[3] Soon after, reports appeared of this procedure being attempted in other countries, particularly Austria, Australia, and England.[4]

CIs became commercially available in 1975. In the relatively brief period that has followed their introduction, CI engineering has progressed from single electrode to multiple-electrode designs that are activated by increasingly sophisticated speech processors.[5]

The earliest CI introduced a single electrode into the base of the cochlea. Although these devices provided some significant benefits, the advent of the multiple-electrode models produced such superior results that they have largely supplanted the single-electrode approaches.

Bioethical questions about implanting young children persist, although the emotions they arouse have faded from prominence.[6] Nonetheless, questions continue to evoke discussion, both domestically and internationally.[7,8]

The flood of research and the wide distribution of CI technology attest to the severity of the condition it addresses and the fruitfulness of the research that has addressed it. As the following indicates, however, efforts to improve the technology continue apace.

## THE CI SYSTEM

The three versions of CIs available in the United States—Nucleus, Advanced Bionics, and Med-El Cochlear Implant Systems—are similar in structure and operation. The following descriptions of the CI apply broadly to all CIs being used in the United States.

### Components

All CIs consist of a battery-powered chain of components that pass the sound input from one component to the other:

- The microphone reacts to sounds in the environment.
- The speech processor selectively responds to the sounds it receives from the microphone. It filters the sounds by converting them to a digital waveform that avoids channel interactions common to analog transmission.[9]
- The transmitter converts the processor's output into electrical impulses.
- The electrodes that are embedded in the auditory portion of the eighth nerve are activated by the impulses it receives from the transmitter. When the auditory nerve has sufficient active fibers, it passes the electrical stimulation to the brain where it can be perceived as sound.

Signals pass from the external apparatus to the electrodes by either transcutaneous or percutaneous links. The former attaches magnetically to a companion coil implanted in the temporal bone and transmission is via radio frequency. Wires from this connection lead to the electrodes in the cochlea. The percutaneous connection plugs directly into the electrode array.

A newer surgical option—minimally invasive cochlear implantation—has been attempted. It differs from previous efforts in that it involves a much smaller scalp flap than conventional CI, which supposedly reduces infection among its benefits.[10]

## Electronic Features

The CI can enable patients to remain in auditory contact with the environment—that is, to be aware of sounds arising around them without much discrimination between them—or it may fully attain the ultimate goal—to enable users to hear and understand speech—or both to some degree. With more specific inputs possible from the additional electrodes, speech discrimination improves greatly over the single-electrode CI.

## HOW THE CI WORKS

The CI system does not provide normal hearing. It is not a hearing aid. It does not "cure" deafness. The CI creates a digital representation of sounds received within a defined bandwidth. When performing optimally, the CI provides stimuli to which patients can react as *if they heard*. However, when the CI is inactivated, the implanted individual remains deaf.[11]

To point out CI's limitations does not deny its sizable contributions to hearing rehabilitation. Providing hearing contact with the environment alone appears to justify its risk and expense. In addition, most deaf people find the CI improves their ability to speechread and improves their voice qualities, probably due to better feedback from their speech.[12]

## IMPLANT VARIATIONS

A CI variation is the hybrid that has been designed for persons with high-frequency hearing losses that cannot be helped by conventional amplification and whose low-frequency hearing is normal or is mildly affected. Using a short electrode can leave low-frequency hearing intact.[13]

Identical to the CI in its external construction, the hybrid device uses a shortened cochlear implant electrode array that is inserted 10 to 20 cm into the cochlea versus 20 to 30 cm for a conventional implant.[14-16] The intent is to improve high-frequency hearing while preserving the low-frequency hearing. Studies are underway to determine the benefits of this technique.[17,18]

Other alternatives to the CI are the Auditory Brain Implant (ABI) and the Penetrating Auditory Brain Implant (PABI).[19] These are designed for persons whose anatomy obviates the use of a CI; for example, when the auditory nerve has been damaged during removal of an acoustic tumor.[20]

The PABI differs from the hybrid in that its placement of electrodes is bifurcated, with one portion positioned in the cochlear nucleus at the base of the brainstem and the other in an adjacent region with the intent of providing better pitch discrimination. The results, although not as beneficial as those for the conventional CI, show substantial gains in sound awareness, speech reading, and speech perception.[21]

## CANDIDACY

Experts convened by the American Speech-Language-Hearing Association posed three questions to guide the decision whether or not to implant:

- Is physical implantation of the device possible and/or advisable given the medical status of the patients?
- Is it likely that an individual will receive more communication benefit from a cochlear implant than from a hearing aid or, alternatively, from no hearing prosthesis at all?
- Do the necessary supports exist in the individual's psychological, family, educational, and rehabilitative situ-

ation to keep a cochlear implant working and integrate it into the patient's life? If not, can they be developed?[22]

These questions do not exhaust those that confront the CI team, when confronting candidates.[23] See "The Cochlear Implant Team" below.

## Anatomic and Physiologic Considerations

Critical to the decision to implant is the condition of the candidate's auditory anatomy and physiology. All deaf people cannot be implanted effectively. Some lack a sufficiently functional auditory nerve. Others have anomalies in inner-ear structure that would rule out a CI, such as cochlear ossification. Functional magnetic-resonance imaging (MRI) can assess residual hearing in children, and this technique may also be useful in predicting success of CI.[24]

A potentially negative indication is so much bony growth in the inner ear that electrodes cannot be introduced into the cochlea. When ossification, which may result from bacterial meningitis, requires extensive drilling to create space for the electrode array, the results are less satisfactory than in the typical case. Also, the potential arises for complications involving the facial nerve.[25] However, if an adequate number of electrodes can be partially inserted and activated, the results may justify implantation.[26] Even children with inner-ear malformations may enjoy a favorable outcome from CI.[27]

The etiologic basis of deafness seems to be a factor in determining the CI's benefits. For example, when deafness due to MYH9 genetic mutation was compared to that due to DFNA17—the former in an American family and the latter in an Australian family—the result favored the use of CI with the DFNA17 deafness.[28] However, children with GJB2 deafness compared to those without this genetic anomaly did not differ in the results of their implantations.[29] Some relations between outcomes and genetic causes of deafness have also appeared with connexin mutations.[30,31]

The management of Neurofibromatosis Type II favors ABI and PABI over conventional CI. The surgical removal of the bilateral tumors that grow on the vestibular portions of nVIII often results in severing the auditory portions of the nerve, rendering a CI ineffective. The ABI and PABI can provide useful stimulation when the CI cannot.

For patients with "ski-slope" auditory configurations, the choice of a CI introduces the risk of losing some of the normal to near-normal hearing for the low frequencies in return for stimulation of the absent or diminished high-frequency responses —something that some patients are reluctant to change. A partial CI, in which insertion of the electrodes remain at the base of the cochlea, can provide a less risky alternative, as it does not destroy all or portions of the hair cells providing the low-frequency hearing.[32]

A case of misdirected implantation highlights another possible complication. Following the patient's complaints of vertigo, a postoperative CT scan found stimulation misdirected to the vestibular portion of the inner ear. It was removed and replaced with a properly placed CI, giving the patient a completely satisfactory outcome.[33]

Studying placement of the CI in situ can be done with MRI without concern about the procedure damaging the CI. A study of 16 implants using a 1.5-Tesla MRI on subjects with Cochlear Nucleus (R) 24 implants did not result in significant loss of magnetization of the CI's internal magnet and did not displace the magnet when external compression dressing was applied.[34]

## Age and Patient's Health

Age does not appear to be a determining factor in the decision to implant or not. As a general rule, the earlier the CI is applied, the better the results; hence, children as young as one year have been successfully implanted.[35]

Concern about their changing skull size and shape has largely been diminished, if not completely eliminated, by procedures to provide slack in the connections to the electrode, thus ensuring that the skull's growth will not displace them.

At the other end of the age continuum, the health of patients, not their chronologic ages, appears critical. Consonant-vowel-consonant word scores and sentence recognition may measure some predictability of adult CI performance.[36]

## Onset of Deafness

The time between the onset of deafness and implantation is a major determiner of the CI's effectiveness—but not in the decision to implant it. The shorter the period of auditory deprivation, the better the results.

## BILATERAL IMPLANTATION

Studies have been made on the extent to which bilateral CIs improve speech understanding and sound localization.[37-39] To date, results appear to favor bilateral implantation, especially in noise, and in improved sound localization.[40] However, diverse results have been reported.[41] To some extent, localization by adults with bilateral CI relates to electrode distribution and spectrum frequency.[42] Other factors also play a part in determining the benefits of bilateral CIs.[43,44] Some adults' localization in noise improved for some but not for other participants in one study, with similarly mixed results for speech perception.[45]

The question of whether a CI can be combined with a hearing aid to achieve optimal results remains open.[46] A further question that begs for investigation is whether results from such a combination would differ between adults and children.

## THE COCHLEAR IMPLANT TEAM

Answering these questions usually involves a professional team that consists of, at a minimum, an otologic surgeon and an audiologist, and should include one or more speech-language pathologists, educators, psychologists, radiologists, and social workers.

# LEARNING TO USE CI

Because the CI does not transmit sound—it transmits a sound analog—the patient must learn to use the instrument's input. For example, when first activated, postlingually deafened adults often report confusion over what they are "hearing." A usual response to initial stimulation is that "speech sounds like Donald Duck." Typically, such reactions for persons with prior hearing experience quickly dissipate in favor of treating stimulations as if they were customary sounds.

Persons who are prelingually deaf do not depend on their auditory memories to interpret the incoming stimulations. When they acquire a CI, they likely undergo a learning process similar to that of a newborn child. Properly guided, they can learn to interpret speech and environmental sounds reliably. Their earlier dependence for communication on sign language and speech reading can be assets to adjusting to the CI and the access it provides to sounds, especially speech that they may not previously have had.[47]

Educators continue to investigate procedures for assisting patients to adapt to CI. Early approaches followed auditory-training programs, which have limitations for those who are prelingually deaf and may be inappropriate for some who are postlingually deafened. The conditions for early deafened versus late-deafened patients suggest that individual approaches are needed to obtain optimal effectiveness.

Selecting an educational setting for children with CI involves choices that are not always evident. Although no one facility will accommodate all such children equally well, some approaches appear broadly applicable, foremost being a nurturing academic environment that fosters speech and language development. Such an environment should include personnel experienced in managing children with CI, availability of audiologic support, and a school administration and staff that is willing to permit and to employ flexibility in the curriculum. Given these features, a child is likely to derive maximum benefit from a CI.[48,49]

Postlingually deaf persons already have learned responses to sounds, so they tend to match the CI stimulation to past experiences. Some find this easier than others, usually in relation to their intellectual status. Others find that the CI input only allows them to be aware of environmental sounds—a modest improvement over deafness but one that most appreciate and will not give up, even if their CI does not provide intelligible speech through the ear alone.

Rehabilitation efforts for all CI users should be directed to such activities of daily living as using the telephone. Unlike hearing aids, the CI does not have a telephone switch. The CI users must learn to identify compatible instruments and adapt to them.[50] The CI user should learn techniques to take full advantage of the combined instrumentation.

Additional instruction is needed to deal with noisy situations and attending to lectures and entertainments in which the CI user is distant from the sound source. Dealing with unfavorable signal-to-noise ratios is almost as much a problem for CI users as for hearing-aid users.

## EVALUATING CI PERFORMANCE

Comparisons between hearing aids and CIs increasingly make use of evidence-based outcomes. Like hearing aids, CIs do not benefit all deaf people equally: performance with these instruments varies greatly from person to person. The future of hearing research will depend on what questions are asked about each approach to hearing rehabilitation.[51]

### Age and Results

For young, born-deaf children, the task is learning to make use of a new sensory input. The time for this adaptation can extend upward of a year, with continuous improvement over an even longer period of time. However, for a majority of the reported cases, speech and language improvements—particularly speech intelligibility—often appear in the first months postactivation. Studies of speech, language, and reading consistently show that children who are implanted during the preschool years or early school years benefit from the auditory experience provided by these devices.[52,53]

A 10-year study of CI performance found no correlation with duration of deafness in adults prior to implantation. During the study period, scores on word recognition remained stable and device failures and explantings were nil.[54]

A study of children with CI's classroom performances compared with non-hearing-impaired children found those with CI did significantly less well. However, age at implantation and duration of deafness contributed the most to the variability of results among children with CIs.[55] Another study found 4 of 5 children implanted before they were 3 years of age used phonological processes more than expected from normative children of comparable age.[56]

Another factor to consider with regard to acquiring reading skills is the child's phonological-processing skills with a CI. One study found accuracy of nonword repetition correlated with nonword reading ability, suggesting that such practice can positively influence word learning.[57]

The difficulties associated with evaluating children decrease as their ages and language abilities increase, so a broad variety of procedures should be available to the cochlear implant team, including parental and teacher reports. Standard audiologic examinations suitable to the children assess sensitivity to sounds, and when appropriate, speech reception can be assessed with tests like the Infant-Toddler Meaningful Auditory Integration Scale and Early Speech Perception Test.[58-60]

After activation of their implants, adult patients' sensitivities to sounds are determined by a standard audiologic examination. To assess their ability to discriminate speech, they are further tested with open-set and spoken-word recognition protocols, monosyllabic-word tests, and sentence-recognition in noise.

## Age at Implantation

For deaf children, evidence suggests that speech perception relates significantly to age at implantation. That study, however, did not find similar relationships between age at implantation and speech production, reading, or language.[61]

A sample of 749 patients was tested after CI implantations. Based on monosyllabic speech-recognition scores, their age at implantation had less predictive power than the durations of their deafness and of their residual speech recognition.[62]

## Results:  Special Populations

Studies of multiply disabled children have found that they benefit from CI, although progressing more slowly and often to a lesser degree.[63] Speech and language performance may differ for groups of various disabilities (see individual disorders in Section 1).

## Cost-Utility Evaluation

The CI's cost-utility compares favorably with medical and surgical interventions that are commonly covered by third-party payers in the United States today, according to one study.[64] A prospective study reached essentially the same conclusion.[65]

Initial costs of a CI range upward of $45,000, which does not include educational expenses and long-term upkeep. For many potential CI candidates, third-party involvement is economically essential. So far, the increased demand for CIs has not resulted in hoped-for reductions in costs of the instrument and of implantation. However, Medicaid, Medicare, and most insurance providers now reimburse some portion of the costs of the surgery and of the device. In the case of employed adults, allowances need be made for time away from work and similar expenses during and immediately following surgery.[66]

## SIDE AND LONG-TERM EFFECTS

All surgery poses some risks and discomforts.[67] To date, reports of surgical mishaps associated with implantation are infrequent.[68]

Swelling around the surgical site usually subsides about 45 days postsurgery, at which time the CI can be activated. However, a recent study reports no danger to the CI from the surgical approach taken (coblation or monopolar electrosurgery).[69]

Preserving residual hearing is also a consideration. The surgical approach and skill of the surgeon determine the extent that result is achievable.[70]

There will be some postoperative restrictions on lengthy immersion in water—as in showering and swimming. Magnetic-resonance imaging (MRI) is usually not allowed because of possible damage to the CI's functioning, although these restrictions may be changing, but, a recent study did not confirm that contention (see ref. 24 above).[71]

### Infections

Infections may be a concern for parents. So far, parents should be assured that the CI does not interfere with treatments for their children's ear infections.[72] The rate of all infections among individuals with CI has been estimated to be between 1 and 2%.

The U.S. Food and Drug Administration (FDA) has undertaken an investigation of possible connections between CI and meningitis. It studied 4,264 children and found 26 had had bacterial meningitis, about 25 times the expected frequency of this infection.[73] In particular, a risk of bacterial meningitis has been noted for CI patients who have a CI from Advanced Bionics; however, its positioner—which may have been the cause of some cases of meningitis—has been redesigned to eliminate that potential hazard. The FDA has outlined steps that should be taken to protect children with CI against bacterial meningitis and other ear infections.

Investigators found a complication rate for minimally invasive CI to be 12.5%, based on the review of 176 records from the University of Texas Health Science Center, San Antonio. Seven patients had major complications—requiring hospitalization or further surgery or involved meningitis and facial-nerve injury—and 15 had minor complications that could be managed conservatively on an ambulatory basis.[74]

## OTHER CONSIDERATIONS

Teenagers who are highly conscious of appearances may reject their implants' external features, rendering them objectionable to useless. They may resent that the CI limits such activities as swimming and contact sports. With counseling, however, such reactions can be overcome and the CI's benefits retained.

It does not appear to matter which ear receives the implant, providing both ears are free of structural abnormalities. What is more likely to be definitive is the status of residual spiral ganglion cells (as noted above).

Patients with CI can expect to visit audiologists throughout their lives, in order to reprogram the system and change speech processors, as their individual conditions require. Changes in their external processors only involve some inconvenience and small expense, and surgery to replace implants does not appear to preclude successful use of CI. A study of 28 children whose CIs were revised concluded that the majority of them recovered their former level of performance.[75]

Some early concerns about the long-term reliability of CI do not appear to be justified; for example, doubts about resistance to corrosion of CI's electrodes has proved unnecessary. Reimplantation due to failure of the electrodes, migration of the unit, and other causes appears seldom to be needed, although occurrences may increase as more surgeons do more implanting. However, if the CI fails for whatever reason, it can be replaced, and experience has shown that the replacement is apt to perform as well or better than the one it replaces.[76]

# THE FUTURE

Because of the impact that CI has had on hearing rehabilitation, research can be expected to continue into the above and related areas. A variety of directions in which such studies can be anticipated include the categories mentioned above and related questions, such as higher levels of neural control.[77] CI investigations may provide models for all audiologic research.[78]

The means of delivering stimulation to the cochlea is being researched. Animal studies compared laser to low-energy electric stimulation and found the former superior because the laser delivers more precise stimulation than the electric transmission, which tends to spread beyond the appropriate nerve cells. Possible tissue damage to the cochlea from lasers' heat needs to be studied, along with the effectiveness of combining light and electric stimulation.[79]

Another possible development is a completely implanted CI. That such an innovation can be achieved in the near term requires extensive research, but it is a developmental avenue being given consideration.[80]

# REFERENCES

1. Djourno A, Eyries C. Prosthese auditive par excitation electrique a distance du nerf sensorial a l'aide d'un bobinage inclus a demeure. *Press Med.* 1957;35:14-17.
2. Simmons FB, Epley JM, Lummis RC. Auditory nerve: electrical stimulation in man. *Science.* 1965;148 (3666):104-106.
3. House WF. Cochlear implants. *Ann Otol Rhinol Laryngol.* 1976;85(3, pt 2, suppl 27):1-23.
4. Schein JD. Cochlear implants and the education of deaf children. *Am Ann Deaf.* 1984;129:324-332.
5. Gantz B, Tyler RS, Abbas PJ, et al. Evaluation of five different cochlear implant designs: audiologic assessment and predictors of performance. *Laryngoscope.* 1988;98:1100-1106.
6. Cohen NL. The ethics of cochlear implants in young children. *Am J Otol.* 1994;15:1-2.

7. L Komesaroff, ed. *Surgical Consent: Bioethics and Cochlear Implantation*. Washington, DC: Gallaudet University Press; 2007.

8. Luterman D. Technology and early childhood deafness. *ASHA Leader*. 2007;12:1.

9. Ricketts T, Grantham DW, D'Hawse PD, et al. Cochlear implant speech processor placement and compression effects on sound sensitivity and interaural level difference. *J Am Acad Audiol*. 2006;17(2):133–140.

10. Stratigouleas ED, Perry BP, King SM, et al. Complication rate of minimally invasive cochlear implantation. *Otolaryngol Head Neck Surg*. 2006;135: 383–386

11. Luterman D. Children with hearing loss: reflections on the past 40 years. *ASHA Leader*. 2004;9:6–7, 18–21.

12. Cohen NL. Cochlear implant surgery. What parents need to know. In: Estabrooks W, ed. *Cochlear Implants for Kids*. Washington, DC: Alexander Graham Bell Association; 1998.

13. Yoo WN, Turner CW, Gantz BJ. Stability of low-frequency residual hearing in patients who are candidates for combined acoustic plus electric hearing. *J Speech Lang Hear Res*. 2004; 49:1085–1090.

14. Ross M. Different kinds of cochlear implants: Auditory, penetrating and hybrid. *Hearing Loss*. 2006;27(3):24–28.

15. Turner CW, Gantz BJ, Vidal C, et al. Speech recognition in noise for cochlear implant listeners: benefits of residual acoustic hearing. *J Acoust Soc Am*. 2004;115:1729–1735.

16. Gifford RH, Shallop JK. Hearing preservation in patients with a cochlear implant. *ASHA Leader*. 2007;12(14): 15, 17, 34

17. Gantz BJ, Turner CW. Combining acoustic and electrical speech processing: Iowa/Nucleus hybrid implant. *Acta Otolaryngol*. 2004;124:344–347.

18. Gantz BJ, Turner C, Gfeller KE. Acoustic plus electric speech processing: preliminary results of a multicenter clinical trial of the Iowa/Nucleus hybrid implant. *Audiol Neurol*. 2006; 11(suppl 1):63–68.

19. Otto S, Shannon RV, Brackman DF, et al. The multichannel auditory brainstem implant: performance in 20 patients. *Otolarygol Head Neck Surg*. 1998;118:291–303.

20. Gantz BJ, Meyer TA. Auditory brain stem implants. In: Cummings CW, ed. *Otolaryngology: Head and Neck Surgery*. Philadelphia, Pa: Mosby; 2005:3845–3854.

21. Auditory brainstem implant. Retrieved July 2007 from http://hei.org/news/facts/abifact.htm

22. Working Group on Cochlear Implants, American Speech and Hearing Association. *Technical Report: Cochlear Implants.* Washington, DC; 2004:1–35.

23. Zwolan TA. Selection of cochlear implant candidates. In: Waltzman S, Cohen N, eds. *Cochlear Implants.* New York, NY: Thieme; 2006:57–68.

24. Patel AM, Cahill LD, Ret J, et al. Functional magnetic resonance imaging of hearing-impaired children under sedation before cochlear implantation. *Arch Otolaryngol Head New Surg.* 2007;133(7):677–683.

25. Niparko JK, Oviatt D, Coker N, et al. Facial nerve stimulation with cochlear implant. *Otolaryngol Head Neck Surg.* 1991; 104:826–830.

26. Kemink J, Zimmerman-Phillips S, Kileny PR, et al. Auditory performance of children with cochlear ossification and partial implant insertion. *Laryngoscope.* 1992;102:1002–1005.

27. Kim L-S, Jeong S-W, Huh M-J, et al. Cochlear implantation in children with inner ear malformations. *Ann Otol Rhinol Laryngol.* 2006;115(3):205–216.

28. Hildebrand MS, de Silva MG, Gardnes RJM et al. Cochlear implants for DFNA17 deafness. *Laryngoscope.* 2006;116: 2211–2215.

29. Propst EJ, Prapsin BC, Stockley TL, et al. Auditory responses in cochlear implant users with and without GJB2 deafness. *Laryngoscope.* 2005;110:317–327.

30. Sinnathuray AR, Toner JG, Clarke-Lyttle J, et al. Connexin 26 (GJB2) gene-related deafness and speech intelligibility after cochlear implantation. *Otol Neurotol.* 2004;25(6):935–942.

31. Lustig LR, Lin D, Venick V, et al. MDGJB2 gene mutations in cochlear implant recipients: prevalence and impact on outcome. *Arch Otolaryngol Head Neck Surg.* 2004;130:541–546.

32. Gantz BJ, Perry BP, Rubinstein JT. Cochlear implants. In: Canalis R, Lambert P, eds. *The Ear: Comprehensive Otology.* Philadelphia, Pa: Lippincott Williams & Wilkins; 2000:633–645.

33. Tange RA, Grolman W, Maat A. Intracochlear misdirected implantation of a cochlear implant. *Acta Otolaryngol.* 2006;126: 650–652.

34. Gubbels SP, McMenomey SO. Safety study of the Cochlear Nucleus (R) 24 device with internal magnet in the 1.5 Tesla magnetic resonance imaging scanner. *Laryngoscope.* 2006; 116(6):865–871.

35. Geers AE. Speech, language, and reading skills after early cochlear implantation. *Arch Otolaryngol Head Neck Surg.* 2004;130:634–638.

36. Gomaa NA, Rubinstein JT, Lowder MW, et al. Residual speech perception and cochlear implant performance in postlingually deafened adults. *Ear Hear.* 2003;24(6):539–544.

37. Tyler RS, Gantz BJ. Rubinstein JT, et al. Three-month results with bilateral cochlear implants. *Ear Hear.* 2002;23:80–89.

38. Gantz BJ, Tyler RS, Rubenstein JT, et al. Binaural cochlear implants placed during the same operation. *Otol Neurotol.* 2002;23:169–180.

39. Tyler RS, Dunn CC. Witt SA, et al. Update on bilateral cochlear implantation. *Curr Opin Otolaryngol Head Neck Surg.* 2003;11:388–393.

40. Van Hoesel RJM, Tyler RS. Speech perception, localization, and lateralization with bilateral cochlear implants. *J Acoust Soc Am.* 2003;113(3):1617–1630.

41. Tyler RS, Noble W, Dunn C, et al. Some benefits and limitations of binaural cochlear implants and our ability to measure them. *Int J Audiol.* 2006;45(suppl 1):113–119.

42. Dunn C, Tyler RS, Witt SA, et al. Frequency and electrode contributions to localization in bilateral cochlear implants. In: Miyamoto R, ed. *Cochlear Implants.* Amsterdam: Elsevier; 2004:443–446.

43. Tyler RS, Preece JP, Wilson BS, et al. Distance, localization and speech perception pilot studies with bilateral cochlear implants. In: Kubo T, Takahasi Y, Iwaki T, eds. *Cochlear Implants—An Update.* The Hague, Netherlands: Kugler Publications; 2002: 517–522.

44. Noble W, Tyler R, Dunn C, et al. Binaural hearing has advantages for cochlear implant users also. *Hear J.* 2005;58(11): 56–64.

45. Dunn CC, Tyler RS, Witt SA. Benefit of wearing a hearing aid on the unimplanted ear in adult users of a cochlear implant. *J Speech Lang Hear Res.* 2005;48:668–680.

46. Tyler RS, Parkinson AJ, Wilson BS, et al. Patients utilizing a hearing aid and a cochlear implant: speech perception and localization. *Ear Hear.* 2002;23(2):98–105.

47. Nussbaum D, LaPorta R, Hinger J. *Cochlear Implants and Sign Language: Putting It All Together (identifying practices for educational settings).* Washington, DC: Gallaudet University Laurent Clerc National Deaf Education Center; 2002:1–89.

48. Zwolan TA. Cochlear implants. In: Katz J, ed. *Handbook of Clinical Audiology.* 5th ed. Philadelphia, Pa: Lippincott Williams & Wilkins; 2002:740–757.

49. Chute PM, Nevins ME. Cochlear implants in children. In: Valente M, Hosford-Dunn H, Roeser RJ, eds. *Audiology: Treatment.* New York, NY: Thieme; 2000.

50. Tearney L. Telephone options for cochlear implant users. *Hear Loss.* 2006;27(2):26–30.

51. Fabry D. Creating the evidence: lessons from cochlear implants. *J Am Acad Audiol.* 2005;16:515–522.

52. Marangos N, Stecker M, Sollman WP, et al. Stimulation of the cochlear nucleus with multichannel auditory brainstem implants and long- term results. *J Laryngol Otol.* 2000;27: 27–31.

53. Dettman SJ, Leigh JR, Dowell RC, et al. The narrow window: early cochlear implant use. *Volta Voices.* 2007;14(6):28–31.

54. Ruffin CV, Tyler RS, Witt SA, et al. Long-term performance of Clarion 1.0 cochlear implant users. *Laryngoscope.* 2007; 1183–1190.

55. Damen GWJA, van den Oever-Goltstein MHL, Langereis MC, et al. Classroom performance of children with cochlear implants in mainstream education. *Ann Otol Rhinol Laryngol.* 2006; 115(7):542–552.

56. Buhler HC, Thomasis BD, Chute P, et al. An analysis of phonological process use in young children with cochlear implants. *Volta Rev.* 2007;107(1):55–74.

57. Dillon CM, Pisoni DB. Nonword repetition and reading skills in children who are deaf and have cochlear implants. *Volta Rev.* 2006;106:121–146.

58. Allum JH, Greisiger R, Straubhaar S, et al. Auditory perception and speech identification in children with cochlear implants tested with the EARS protocol. *Br J Audiol.* 2000;34:293–303.

59. Zimmerman-Phillips S, Robbins AM, Osberger MJ. Assessing cochlear implant benefit in very young children. *Ann Otol, Rhinol Laryngol*. 2000;185:42–43.

60. Moog JS, Geers AE. *Early Speech Perception Test for Profoundly Hearing-Impaired Children*. St. Louis, Mo: Central Institute for the Deaf; 1990.

61. Geers AE. Speech language, and reading skills after early cochlear implantation. *JAMA*. 2004;291(19):2378–2380.

62. Leung J, Wang N-Y, Yeagle JD, et al. Predictive models for cochlear implantation in elderly candidates. *Arch Otolaryngol Head Neck Surg*. 2005;131:1049–1053.

63. Waltzman SB, Scalchunes V, Cohen NL. Performance of multiply handicapped children using cochlear implants. *Am J Otol*. 2000;21:321–335.

64. Cheng AK, Niparko JK. Cost-utility of the cochlear implant in adults. A meta-analysis. *Arch Otolaryngol Head Neck Surg*. 1999;125:1214–1218.

65. Palmer CS, Niparko JK, Wyatt JR, et al. A prospective study of the cost-utility of the multichannel cochlear implant. *Arch Otolaryngol Head Neck Surg*. 1999;125:1221–1228.

66. Low levels of insurance reimbursement impede access to cochlear implants. Retrieved September 2006 from http://www.rand.org/pubs/research_briefs/RB4532-1/index1.html

67. Cohen NL, Roland JT. Complications of cochlear implant surgery. In: Waltzman SB, Cohen NL, eds. *Cochlear Implants*. New York, NY: Thieme; 2006:126–132.

68. Migirov L, Yakirevitch A, Kronenberg J. Surgical and medical complications following cochlear implantation: comparison of two surgical approaches. *ORL*. 2006;68:213–219.

69. Antonelli P, Baratelli R. Cochlear implant integrity after adenoidectomy with coblation and monopolar electrosurgery. *Am J Otolaryngol*. 2006;28(1):9–12.

70. Turner C, Gantz B. Preservation of residual acoustic hearing in cochlear implantation. In: Miyamoto RT, ed. *Cochlear Implants. Proceedings of the VIII International Cochlear Implant Conference,* Indianapolis, Ind, May 10–13, 2004. Philadelphia, Pa: Elsevier; 2004:243–246.

71. Balkany TJ, Gantz BJ. Medical and surgical considerations in cochlear implants. In: Cummings C, Flint PW, Haughey BH,

et al, eds. *Otolaryngol Head and Neck Surgery*. Philadelphia, Pa: Elsevier; 2004.

72. Luterman, D. Counseling parents about cochlear implants. *ASHA Leader.* 2003;8:6-7, 20-21.

73. Cochlear implants and bacterial meningitis. Retrieved February 2006 from http://www.fda.gov/fdac/features/2003/603_implant.html

74. Stratigouleas E, Perry B, King S, et al. Complication rate of minimally invasive cochlear implantation. *Otolaryngol Head Neck Surg.* 2007;135(3):383-387.

75. Fayad JN, Eisenberg LS, Gillinger M, et al. Clinical performance of children following revision surgery for a cochlear implant. *Otolaryngol Head Neck Surg.* 2006;134:379-384.

76. Kirk KI, Miyamoto RT, Lento CI, et al. Effects of age at implantation in young children. *Ann Otol Rhinol Laryngol.* 2002; 111:69-73.

77. Wilson BS, Lawson DS, Muller JM, et al. Cochlear implants: some likely next steps. *Ann Rev Biomed Eng.* 2003;5:207-249.

78. Jerger J. Editorial. *J Am Audiol Assoc.* 2006;17(2):1.

79. Izzo AD, Pathria ESJ, Waslsh JT, et al. Selectivity of neural stimulation in the auditory system: a comparison of optic and electric stimuli. *J Biomed Optics.* 2007;12(2):1-7.

80. Cohen NL. Considerations for devising a totally implantable cochlear implant. In: Waltzman S, Cohen N, eds. *Cochlear Implants.* New York, NY: Thieme; 2006:230-232.

# Section 2.3

# *Strategies to Compensate for Hearing Loss*

Educational and psychological approaches have key roles to play in the management of persons with impaired hearing and vestibular functions. The professionals who make up a Hearing Rehabilitation Team (HRT) responsible for patients with hearing losses must be prepared to counsel and educate, as well as to diagnose, treat, and refer, when indicated.[1]

Dealing successfully with hearing loss involves much more than its diagnosis and initial treatment. It requires professional concern for its meaning and providing counseling to resolve the feelings that it arouses. It means allowing frequent revisits to reprogram any prostheses, be they hearing aids or cochlear implants. It also should involve establishing a relationship with the patient to provide for changes in hearing status, which can optimize the success of initial diagnosis and treatment.[2]

## THE HEARING REHABILITATION TEAM (HRT)

A single individual rarely has the range of competencies that are required to conduct the preceding activities successfully.[3] Hence, the HRT should include personnel whose educational preparation and experience qualifies them to perform at least some of the services required by persons with impaired hearing. The HRT consists of audiologists, otologists, speech-language pathologists, psychiatrists, psychologists, and social workers, along with educators, pediatricians, neurologists, other professionals and may include hearing-aid specialists.[4,5]

Different members of the HRT may be assigned to perform the variety of tasks that patient management requires. Within the team, its members must be familiar with the wide variety of assistive equipment that can alleviate or eliminate particular problems faced by persons with hearing loss; for example, assistive-listening devices (ALD) and lights that signal doorbells and telephones are ringing. In addition, one team member must be in a position to integrate all of the information and to present it to the patient.[6]

New technologic versions of established instruments and techniques continually arise, as do reshaping of professions to reflect new approaches to management.[7] One such adaptation is UBI DUO—essentially paired computers that enable one person to read what another person types and to respond in real time.[8] It enables deaf and hard-of-hearing persons to communicate in real time with each other and with normally hearing persons without interpreters or pad and pencil.

## COUNSELING AND EDUCATION

Counseling begins at the first contact with the patient (often a phone call to the audiologist's office) and continues through the duration of patient-therapist relations. Many clinicians consider counseling the most overlooked aspect of the process of fitting amplification.[9] At the same time it is probably the most important professional service the HRT can provide for patients and their families.[10]

### Gaining Acceptance of Amplification

Education and counseling merge at appropriate times in patient-clinician contacts. Patients need information, instruction, and emotional support.[11] Such counseling can lead to improved acceptance of hearing aids and can increase and improve their use.[12,13]

Another factor in gaining consumer acceptance of hearing aids is cosmetic. Suggestions have been made to improve the appropriate use of hearing aids by attention to the instruments' appearance.[14] The trend toward making hearing aids inconspicuous with in-the-ear and open-canal fitting also seems to boost their acceptance.[15]

## Types of Counseling

Counseling may be differentiated by type into informational and affective or emotional.[16] Informational counseling teaches about and provides practice in managing amplification devices and confronting listening challenges. Affective or emotional counseling deals with the psychological adjustment to the hearing loss and its rehabilitation.

## Informational Counseling and Instruction

The HRT provides knowledge that patients need, in order to better adjust to hearing loss and/or vestibular damage. Which members of the team provide which aspects of the counseling depends on their interpersonal skills, available time, and personal preferences.

Hearing-aid orientation introduces the patients to their equipment and instructs them on how to use and care for the prescribed hearing aids, cochlear implants, and other apparatus.[17] The HRT provides fundamentals; for example, inserting the earmold or the in-the-ear hearing aid, manipulating the volume control, and inserting, checking, and removing the battery.

The HRT arranges for patients and their significant others to obtain information that is specific to their situation. Instruction varies depending on patient's age, intellect, and other personal characteristics. It also takes into account the usual surroundings that are likely to influence the effectiveness of amplification, like classrooms, cars, offices, and factories. Patients should be taught how to handle environmental conditions that are presently difficult for hearing aids and cochlear implants to handle, such as distance from the speaker and noisy surroundings (i.e., poor signal-to-noise ratios).[18]

Persons with hearing losses need Instruction in the care and use of amplification instruments, especially those with cognitive limitations. It is essential to arrange follow-up visits to determine how well instruction has been understood and to answer questions that occur to the patient after a period of use. Whether the patients are young children or mature adults, they can be expected to profit from such instruction when it is tailored to their learning abilities and given in their preferred language.[19]

As the patient's companions' and coworkers' cooperation can greatly enhance hearing rehabilitation, HRT informs the patient and the patient's significant others about how they can optimize communication in the presence of noisy surroundings. When feasible and appropriate, such advice may be given to employers, coworkers and teachers.

By offering its resources to patients and significant relations, the HRT provides a valuable resource, one that is especially useful to parents of hearing-impaired children. As some clinicians have urged, the HRT must be knowledgeable about the efficacy of aural habilitation practices and about how to perform required long-term services, because the HRT is often the first, and sometimes the only, professional group that will provide ongoing authoritative information about hearing impairment and appropriate services to persons with impaired hearing.

## Emotional Support

Although factual presentations can sometimes obviate emotional reactions, often they require discussion with a counselor to answer questions: What does the hearing loss mean to the patient? Is it a sign of declining health, of premature aging, of impending death? If hearing loss is unilateral, will it impact on the unaffected ear?

These questions and the underlying emotions vary depending on the patients' ages at onset of their hearing losses. The counseling requires careful probing and modification of approach based on these factors, among others.[20]

As with any negative alterations in physical condition, hearing loss affects self-image. Counseling can overcome strong negative reactions and is a high priority for the HRT.[21] It has also been shown that patients and parents too often do not recall the information they have been provided, suggesting that the information should be given with emotional support and in written from, if it is to be retained beyond the counseling session.[22,23]

Too often counselors have the notion that they are supposed to do the talking, rather than being sympathetic listeners.[24] In most cases, their educational programs do not prepare them to be effective affective counselors. Their lack of preparation that leads to failure to provide emotional support may underlie complaints patients mistakenly attribute entirely to their hearing aids.

Counseling offers patients an opportunity to vent their fears and unhappiness about their specific listening challenges. Such catharsis not only can relieve the patient, but also may reveal misapprehensions the clinician can address. Overly optimistic expectations can reduce the benefits that would otherwise accrue from amplification.[25] Encountering other patients in auditory-training groups allows patients to share experiences with those with similar problems, which can be reassuring and help overcome pessimism and frustration.[26]

Formal educational preparation can counter clinicians' lack of responsiveness to patients' need for affective counseling.[27] Unfortunately, many educational programs for audiology and otology students do not require it.[28] Courses on how to conduct counseling have found students more likely to respond to affective statements with affective responses and to be more aware of patients' emotional needs. Such research can also address the question of clinicians' limitations in dealing with patients' psychological problems, if any.[29]

As noted in other areas of expertise, the HRT should be aware of its own strengths and weaknesses and, when appropriate, should be prepared to make referrals to other disciplines that are not part of the team. When clinicians have patients with significant affective disorders in addition to their hearing impairments, they should consult with appropriate professionals in the course of hearing rehabilitation.

## Individual Versus Group Counseling

Although counseling is usually thought of as conducted one-on-one, it can be conducted in groups—saving costs and staff time and, some reports suggest, with only a small loss of effectiveness.

Group approaches may be more useful than individual for some adolescents and adults. They may profit from role-playing exercises in which they can learn and practice tactics and strategies for managing frequently encountered problems without generating embarrassment to themselves or hostility in the offenders.[30]

Some patients may begin with one-to-one counseling and then be assigned to a group. Another option is the use of print materials and computer programs, for which see "Tactics and Strategies to Enhance Communication" below.

## Accommodating Patient Differences

Approaches to patients differ, depending on the characteristics of the patient (e.g., age, gender. cultural) and the nature of the condition that brings them to counseling, as well as the individual differences in reactions to hearing loss. Outcomes depend on many factors, leading some authorities to the conclusion that the success of aural rehabilitation is largely a function of individual differences in patients and in the HRT's skills and not the characteristics of the hearing loss.

# TACTICS AND STRATEGIES TO ENHANCE COMMUNICATION

Hearing rehabilitators have recognized that amplification alone —regardless of how superior its electroacoustical characteristics—will not facilitate a complete return to communication success for every patient. They recognize the need for systematic programs of hearing rehabilitation for significant numbers of new hearing-aid users and the need for additional tactics and equipment.

The Listening and Communication Enhancement Program (LACE) is an interactive, computerized training program designed for home use.[31] A small study suggests that with the establishment of realistic short-term goals, listening skills can be improved.[32]

Researchers have tested the effects of adaptive computer-controlled syllable-identification training on nonsense-syllable-test performance of new and experienced hearing-aid users. The training administered over an 8-week period produced large improvements in syllable identification for both the new and experienced hearing-aid users.[33] Training-related improvement was generalized to connected speech and to untrained voices, and it was maintained on retention tests.

# HEARING AND SPEECH CONSERVATION

The HRT should confer with patients about poor lifestyle habits that can affect all sensory functions and should recommend actions that will correct them. When such recommendations encounter the patient's strong resistance, they may require referral to a specialist in the area of dysfunction; for example, see discussion above about significant affective disorders.

## Speech Conservation

Speech conservation refers specifically to therapy aimed at preserving or improving speech and voice patterns, especially for those with progressive hearing losses. The HRT's speech-language pathologist can provide both diagnosis and treatment.

## Hearing Conservation

To optimize hearing functions, patients should seek prompt treatment for ear and upper-respiratory infections, diabetes, and hypertension. Eliminating smoking and other debilitating habits are also well advised. Noise avoidance is of particular importance to conserving hearing. Patients should limit exposure to loud, intense, and prolonged noises and receive information about hearing-protective devices, in order to preserve their remaining hearing ability.

Although these suggestions are easily made, they may be difficult for the patient to implement. Nonetheless, their place remains high in the hearing rehabilitation program for their obvious importance to maintaining hearing and counterbalancing patients' exclusive focus on their diminished hearing capacity. The HRT should find measures that support these lifestyle recommendations.

## SURGERY AND MEDICATION

Prescribing amplification may not always be appropriate. When the cause of the hearing loss is in the middle ear and the cochlea is normal or near-normal, surgery may correct the disease or malformation, restoring normal to near-normal hearing.

If the hearing loss is caused by an acute infection, medication to cure it can usually return hearing to normal. In both of these instances, the result of correcting the malformation and/or eliminating the infection can usually result in restoring normal to near-normal hearing and giving relief from tinnitus.

Even removal of impacted cerumen can often restore hearing and eliminate or alleviate tinnitus. Thus, amplification is not always the proper response to a hearing loss, particularly when the loss is conductive. It is, however, the most appropriate and frequently prescribed correction for sensorineural hearing loss.

# COMMUNICATION SUPPLEMENTATION

Developing the ability to make use of extra-auditory cues can be useful and, for some patients, essential. The HRT should introduce additional measures that can supplement the rehabilitation program and should be in a position to discuss them when it believes patients are ready to learn about them.

## Speech Reading (or Lip Reading)

Speech reading is preferred over lip reading, although the two terms are often used interchangeably. The former indicates that more than differentiating lip shapes is involved in the process of supplementing oral communication with visual clues.

Successful speech reading depends on context and speaker's posture as well as on lip shapes. It is limited by the many English homonyms, like *time* and *dime*, whose lip shapes are identical. Because it is an inexact form of communication, it has been referred to as "lip-guessing," a humorous term that conveys a sober point.[34]

Classes and individual tutoring in speech reading are available in most urban areas. They can be located by contacting the American-Speech-Language-Hearing Association and the American Academy of Audiology.

Films and computer programs also offer practice opportunities, but they should be accompanied by listening training. Although speech reading is a useful communication adjunct it does not supplant auditory perception.

Overemphasis on developing speech reading skill may frustrate those patients who do not develop it, and this failure can interfere with other aspects of their rehabilitation. Visual and auditory perception can be integrated and taught as a unified skill.

Despite how long speech reading has been available, research continues on further understanding and improving it. A recent study using a new approach (point-light technique) found biases and misreadings can significantly influence the process.[35]

## Telecommunications

Telephones, television, and other telecommunication devices once difficult or impossible to use by people with impaired hearing are accessible to them through a variety of means, as required by recent federal legislation.[36] Amplifiers built into telephones assist persons with hearing losses, as do hearing aids that can be adapted to use with telephones.[37]

Another approach supplants voice with print. For the telephone, this means using teletypewriters (TTYs) that enable both parties to type their messages and have them reproduced as print at the other end. For deaf-blind persons, a Brailler can be added at the receiving end to reproduce the typed input tactually. Relay systems that interpose a hearing person who speaks what a deaf person types and types what is spoken enable communication with persons and facilities that do not have the necessary transmission equipment.

For large meetings, Computer Assisted Realtime Captioning (CART) provides simultaneous captions of speech. A stenographer records all spoken communication using computer software. The computer then displays it on a computer, video or other screen.[38] For further information contact Hearing Loss Association of America (formerly Self-Help for the Hard of Hearing [SHHH]).[39]

- ■ Contact your local chapter
- ■ Check out, a Web site dedicated to Realtime Captioning

Adding captions to films and television programs to reproduce in print the spoken dialogue has a long history. For deaf and hearing-impaired persons, the application of the technique to television has been a welcome extension. The National Captioning Institute is one of several sources of captioning for movies and television. WGBH, Boston's television station, also has lengthy experience captioning its programs and programs that are distributed nationally. The Americans with Disabilities

Act requires the captioning of emergency announcements on television, but, to a large extent, adding printed versions of speech on other television programming and movies remains optional.

Another means to overcome hearing impairments is to use infrared and hard-wired listening devices to television viewing. Infrared devices are available in some theaters. The receiving amplifiers that translate the transmitted signal are available in theaters that are so equipped. Individuals can also purchase this equipment.

At meetings, an overhead projector can project a hand-written or typed version of what is being spoken, enabling those who cannot hear to follow the discussion in real time.

Relay services are available to persons who cannot hear and telephones and/or whose speaking ability is inadequate. Essentially, these arrangements have an operator who receives the deaf person's messages via TTY, speaks the message to a person whom the deaf person wishes to call, and the operator then relays the spoken message via TTY to the deaf person. Television can facilitate interpreting when the interpreters are distant from their audience. This approach is growing in use as the shortage of interpreters remains.[40]

## Manual Communication

Manual communication can be divided into ad hoc signals (gestures and home signs), formal cues, and sign languages. Although grouped under a single heading, each is a distinctive means of providing communication or communication support.[41]

Ad hoc signals—pointing, gesturing, postures, head nodding, smiles, and grimaces—are commonly used by virtually all persons and in all cultures. Their meanings require no specific instruction, being immediately obvious to those who observe them. They can convey only a narrow range of communication, unless accompanied by speech. Home signs, however, are, as their name implies, signs developed within a family or small group of signers. Understanding them requires specific knowledge held by the small group of signers.

Fingerspelling provides a means of representing words letter-by-letter—an obviously tedious means of communication for all but brief messages. The meaning of particular hand configurations varies, each system unique to a particular country; for example, the British and American versions differ, in that the former uses both hands and the latter only one.[42]

Cued Speech consists of a formal set of hand signals placed at and around the mouth of the speaker to clarify potentially confusing lip shapes.[43] This method has the benefit of focusing attention on speech. Although available in the United States for about 40 years, it is now widely available internationally.[44]

Sign languages are languages that have their own grammar and syntax, separate from the language of the spoken language of the country in which they are used. In the United States, deaf people use American Sign Language (ASL), as well as English. The latter also can be represented by hand-arm-facial expressions, although in that form it lacks the fluidity of ASL. Sign languages have been demonstrated to readily convey actions and ideas in the past, present, and future, as would be expected of true languages.

The notion that there is a universal sign language, however, is mistaken. Each country has its own sign language, distinct from that of other nations and from its spoken language. National sign languages, like spoken languages, also have local variations that can differ widely from the national versions. An Esperanto-like concoction of signs from various places, called Gestuno, has been developed by the World Federation of the Deaf for use at its international conferences. Gestuno lacks grammatic rules and has a limited vocabulary; hence, it is not a sign language but rather is an ad hoc communication adjunct with limited applicability.

Research to better understand how readers of sign language extract information from it find that significant aspects can be derived from relatively minor movements of the body. To facilitate these studies, point-light techniques appear useful.[45]

## DUAL SENSORY IMPAIRMENTS

Dual sensory impairments are relatively rare in the general population.[46] They become increasingly prevalent among persons 70 years of age and older, affecting from 5 to 20%.[47] The reduction in the one distance sense, vision, limits or eliminates some strategies that depend on using it to compensate for hearing loss, especially for activities of daily living.[48] The patient with dual sensory impairments also requires specialized approaches to diagnosis and management.[49] (See Usher syndrome in Section 1.1.)

Despite the severity of dual sensory impairments' effects, most people are unaware of the availability of vision and aural rehabilitation programs. There are procedures and equipment that can be effectively employed.[50]

Being attentive to the vision of all hearing-impaired patients would appear to be an essential component of hearing rehabilitation. The hearing loss may be so great as to obscure a coexisting visual loss. It would be remiss not to suggest that the HRT require visual screening for all patients with hearing loss before completing their rehabilitation plans.

## HEARING EAR DOGS

Service dogs are trained to assist deaf people by alerting them to environmental sounds: doorbells, telephone, whistling teakettles, and much more. The decision to acquire a dog, however, should not be made without considering that the animal requires care as well as giving service.

The considerations that enter into such a decision concern the type of dog, the impact having such a dog will have on the owner's lifestyle, and the time, effort, and expense of maintenance. The owner should also decide if he or she is capable of learning to use the dog properly.[51]

## SELF-HELP GROUPS, GOVERNMENTAL AND VOLUNTARY ORGANIZATIONS

Self-help groups and voluntary organizations provide an adjunct to the HRT's services. The HRT can introduce patients to groups it deems appropriate for them.

The oldest self-help group in the United States is the National Association of the Deaf.[52] In time, several other organizations of and for persons with impaired hearing have arisen; for example, Alexander Graham Association for the Deaf and Hard of Hearing, Association of Late Deafened Adults, and Hearing Loss Association of America (formerly, Self-Help for Hard of Hearing People).

Coalition of Organizations for Accessible Technology (COAT) now has 67 cross-disability members and is open to national, regional and community-based organizations.[53] The National Hearing Conservation Association (NHCA) aims to prevent hearing loss due to noise and other environmental factors. It provides education for professionals and support for research.[54]

Deaf Blind International promotes transnational services for deafblind persons. Among U.S. organizations for deafblind people are the American Printing House for the Blind and the American Foundation for the Blind, whose services extend to deaf blind as well as blind persons. The American Association of the Deaf-Blind serves its members' social needs and represents them before legislatures. Some states also have active facilities that serve deafblind people, like the Alabama Institute for Deaf and Blind and the Alaska Center for Blind and Deaf Adults.

Each state's Division of Vocational Rehabilitation (DVR) should be able to provide the location of voluntary and self-help organizations. States' DVRs also provide funding for education and training of individuals with disabilities.

# BIBLIOTHERAPY

Most of the professional and consumer-advocacy groups produce lists of books, issue periodicals, and maintain Web sites. These resources can add to the hearing-rehabilitation program. Whether to assign them to particular patients, however, is a decision the HRT makes, based on the individual patient's needs and capabilities.

Hearing inventories and questionnaires completed by the patient and the significant other are valuable in assessing the degree of difficulty the patient is experiencing in a variety of real-life situations. The extreme prevalence of self-denial in this population often limits the value of patients' assessments of their difficulties. Completing these instruments helps patients focus on relevant aspect of daily living that then contribute to their realistically facing the deficiencies caused by their hearing losses. (See "The Prefitting Examination" in Section 2.1)

*Access Audiology* is an E-newsletter, written by and for audiologists. It highlights current clinical topics. Members have access to a complete archive of past issues. Experts in audiology, psychology, sociology, and geriatrics offer multidisciplinary views on the aging patient, with emphasis on audiologic service delivery. Clinicians may find some material in it that they might wish to share with patients.[55]

# REFERENCES

1. Crandall CC. An update on counseling instruction within audiology programs. *J Acad Rehabil Audiol.* 1997;30:77–86.
2. Luterman D. The counseling relationship. *ASHA Leader.* 2006; 11(4):8–9, 33.
3. American Speech-Language-Hearing Association. *Knowledge and skills required for the practice of audiological/aural rehabilitation.* Retrieved May 2001 from http://www.asha.org/policy
4. Tye-Murray N. *Foundations of Aural Rehabilitation: Children, Adults, and Their Family Members.* San Diego, Calif: Singular; 1998.

5. Schow RL, Balsara NR, Smedley TC, et al. Aural rehabilitation by ASHA audiologists: 1980–1990. *Am J Audiol.* 1993;2(3): 28–37.

6. Noe CM, McArdle R, Chisholm TH, et al. FM technology use in adults with significant hearing loss. Part I: Candidacy. In: Fabry D, De Johnson CD, eds. *ACCESS: Achieving Clear Communication Employing Sound Solutions.* Chicago, Ill: Phonak; 2004.

7. Jackler RK, Brackmann DE, eds. *Neurotology.* 2nd ed. Philadelphia, Pa: Elsevier; 2005:1047–1069.

8. http://www.scommonline.com/blog

9. *Contemporary Issues in Communication Sciences and Disorders.* Retrieved July 2002 from http://www.nsslha.org/NSSLHA/members/cicsd/cicsd-s02.htm

10. Herzfeld M, English K. Survey of audiology students confirms need for counseling as part of audiologists' training. *Hear J.* 2001;54(5):50–54.

11. Citron D. Appropriate management of psychological barriers to the use of amplification will reduce hearing instrument returns and in-the-drawer hearing aid non-use. Counseling and orientation. In: Valente M, Hosford-Dunn H, Roeser RJ, eds. *Audiology Treatment.* New York, NY: Thieme; 2000.

12. Brooks D. Counseling and its effect on hearing aid use. *Scand Audiol.* 1979;8:101–107.

13. Northern JL, Beyer DM. Reducing hearing aid returns through patient education. *Audiol Today.* 1999;11:10–11.

14. Bartkiw B. Reducing the stigma of deafness—hearing aids with enhanced visual appeal. *Br J Audiol.* 1988;22:167–169.

15. Miller MH, Schein JD. Improving consumer acceptance of hearing aids. *Hear J.* 1987;40(10):25–32.

16. Lucker JR. Finding the right fit: educational audiology takes more than one counseling direction. *ASHA Leader.* 2005; 10(6):18–19.

17. Tyler R, Schum D, eds. *Assistive Devices for Persons with Hearing Impairment.* Boston, Mass: Allyn & Bacon; 1995.

18. Gatehouse S, Naylor G, Elberling C. Benefits from hearing aids in relation to the interaction between the user and the environment. *Int J Audiol.* 2003;42:77–85.

19. Ling D. Advances underlying spoken language development. A century of building on Bell. *Volta Rev.* 1990;92(4):8–20.

20. De Graaf R, Bijl RV. Determinants of mental stress in adults with a severe auditory impairment: differences between prelingual and postlingual deafness. *Psychosom Med.* 2002;64:61-70.

21. Abrams H, Hnath-Chisholm T, Guererrio S, et al. The effects of intervention strategy on self-perception of hearing handicap. *Ear Hear.* 1992;13:371-377.

22. Martin E, Kreuger S, Bernstein M. Diagnostic Information transfer to hearing-impaired adults. *Texas J Audiol Speech Path.* 1990;16(2)29-32.

23. Margolis RH. Boosting memory with informational counseling: helping patients understand the nature of disorders and how to manage them. *ASHA Leader.* 2004;9:10-11, 28.

24. English K, Mendel LL, Rojeski T, et al. Counseling in audiology or learning to listen. *Am J Audiol.* 1999; 8:34-39.

25. Garstecki DC, Erler SF. Counseling older adult hearing instrument candidates. *Hear Rev.* 1997;(suppl 1):14-18.

26. Hawkins D. Effectiveness of counseling-based adult group aural rehabilitation programs: a systematic review of the literature. *J Am Acad Audiol.* 2005;6:485-493.

27. English K. Integrating new counseling skills into existing audiological practices. Retrieved May 2001 from http://www.audiologyonline.com/article/

28. Estabrooks W, ed. *Auditory-Verbal Therapy.* Washington, DC: Alexander Graham Bell Association for the Deaf; 1994.

29. Maki-Torkko EM, Brorsson B, Davis AC, et al. Hearing impairment among adults—extent of the problem and scientific evidence on the outcome of hearing aid rehabilitation. *Scand J Audiol.* 2001;30(suppl 54):8-15.

30. Brickley GJ, Cleaver VC, Bailey S. An evaluation of a group follow-up scheme for new NHS hearing aid users. *Br J Audiol.* 1996;30(5):307-312.

31. Sweetow RW, Palmer CV. Efficacy of individual auditory training in adults: a systematic review of the evidence. *J Am Acad Audiol.* 2005;16:494-504.

32. Sweetow RW, Henderson-Sabe J. The need for and development of an adaptive listening and communication enhancement (LACE) program. *J Am Acad Audiol.* 2006;17:538-558.

33. Stecker GC, Bowman GA, Yund EW, et al. Perceptual training improves syllable identification in new and experienced hearing-aid users. *J Rehab Res Develop.* 2005;43:537-551.

34. Osberger MJ. Speechreading. In: Van Cleve JV, ed. *Gallaudet Encyclopedia of Deaf People and Deafness.* Vol 3. New York, NY: McGraw-Hill; 1987:234–237.

35. Rosenblum LD, Saldana HM. An audiovisual test of kinematic primitives or visual speech perception. *J Exp Psychol: Hum Percept Perform.* 1996;22(2):318–331.

36. Strauss KP. *A New Civil Right: Telecommunications Equality for the Deaf.* Washington, DC: Gallaudet University Press; 2006.

37. Harkins J. Practical information for audiologists on access to wireless telephones. *J Am Acad Audiol.* 2001;12(6):290–295.

38. Computer Assisted Realtime Captioning. Retrieved from http://www.cartinfo.org

39. Hearing Loss Association of America. Access at http://www.shhh.org

40. Stewart DA, Schein JD, Cartwright BE. *Sign Language Interpreting.* 2nd ed. Boston, Mass: Allyn & Bacon; 2004.

41. Schein JD, Stewart DA. *Language in Motion.* Washington, DC: Gallaudet University Press; 1995.

42. Carmel S. *International Hand Alphabet Charts.* Rockville, Md: Studio Printing; 1982.

43. Cornett RO. *Cued Speech Parent Training and Follow-up Programs.* Washington, DC: Bureau of Education for the Handicapped, Department of Health, Education and Welfare; 1972.

44. Beck PH. Cued speech across cultures. *Volta Voices.* 2006; 13(5):26–28.

45. Poizner H, Bellugi U, Lutes-Driscill V. Perception of American sign language in dynamic point-light displays. *J Exp Psychol: Hum Percep Perform.* 1981;7:430–440.

46. Sauerburger D. *Independence Without Sight or Sound.* New York, NY: American Foundation for the Blind; 1993.

47. Brennan M, Su Y, Horowitz A. Longitudinal associations between dual sensory impairment and everyday competence among older adults. *J Rehab Res Develop.* 2006;43(6):777–792.

48. Horowitz A, Reinhardt JP, Brennan M. *Aging and Vision Loss: Experiences, Attitudes and Knowledge of Older Americans.* Final Report submitted to the AARP Andrus Foundation. New York, NY: Arlene R. Gordon Research Institute of the Lighthouse; 1997.

49. Sullivan R, Kramer LC, Hirsch LM. *Audiological Evaluation and Aural Rehabilitation of the Deaf-Blind Adults*. New York, NY: Helen Keller National Center for Deaf-Blind Youth and Adults; 1979.

50. The Helen Keller National Center for Deaf-Blind Youth and Adults is a government-supported resource for information about such aids. For reference materials, consult Deafblind Link and Perkins School for the Blind.

51. Heppner C. A complete guide to man's best friend as a hearing dog. *Hear Loss Mag*. 2007;28(5):10–17.

52. Gannon JR. *Deaf Heritage*. Silver Spring, Md: National Association of the Deaf; 1981.

53. Coalition of Organizations for Accessible Technology (COAT). Access at http://www.coataccess.org

54. National Hearing Conservation Association (NHCA). Access at http://www.hearingconservation.org

55. Retrieved April 2007 from http://www.asha.org/ members/ aud/access-aud-online/default

# SECTION 3

# Demographic, Social, and Economic Aspects

The material in this section regards aspects of hearing and vestibular disorders that apply generally: the geographic, temporal distribution of disorders among populations and the characteristics of those populations that affect significant aspects of their genesis and management. Of further interest are relevant social and economic considerations that, taken together, have programmatic significance as well as some practical applications to the treatment of individual cases.

Size and characteristics of the hearing-impaired population change due to sporadic epidemics, fluctuating birthrates, immigration shifts, and alterations in the composition of the population by age, ethnicity, and gender. The result: estimates of the size and descriptions of the hearing-impaired population vary from place to place and over time.[1]

What can readers do to ensure that they have reliable, up-to-date information relevant to hearing and vestibular disorders? The National Center for Health Statistics (NCHS) provides data that will enable them to stay current about the U.S. population.[2] For other jurisdictions, surfing the Internet may be productive.

Models for gathering such information have been proposed, combining registers of deaf and/or hard-of-hearing people with population surveys.[3,4] Why, then, do we not have more accurate and more current information about hearing loss? Governments have said it is too expensive and invades privacy. However, they conduct ongoing studies of communicable diseases and maintain registers of births, deaths, and driving licenses. In response to the cost argument data-gathering expenses should be balanced against the waste from inaccurate information, which can be far more wasteful of public and private resources than the amounts needed to collect accurate, current data.

Although the size of a statistic will fluctuate over time, trends and relationships between it and other factors tend to be consistent. For that reason—and except to illustrate variability—the following discussion focuses on data that illustrate trends and relationships that have been stable over time, rather than on those for particular years or narrowly defined geographic areas.

## PREVALENCE

Hearing loss is the single most prevalent chronic physical disability in the United States and, possibly, throughout the world. In a given year, more people have common colds than suffer hearing losses, and—over their lifetime—more may suffer a psychiatric illness than a hearing loss. But the common cold is an *acute* affliction and psychiatric conditions are *mental* not physical, illnesses. So hearing loss continues to occupy its primary position in the prevalence of chronic disorders.

### Prevalence over Time

To view some evidence of fluctuations in prevalence rates over time, consider the U.S. Bureau of the Census data on deafness for each decennial year from 1830 to 1930.[5] As seen in Figure 3.1, the rates of deafness more than doubled between a

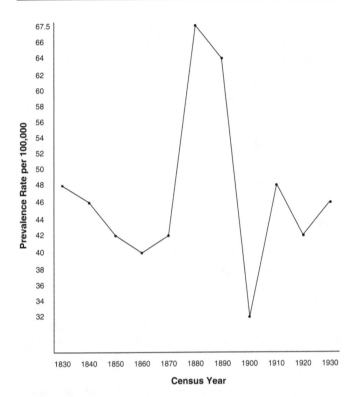

**Figure 3.1.** Prevalence Rates of Deaf-Mutism[a] per 100,000: United States Decennial Census, 1830–1930. ([a]Term used by the Bureau to indicate deafness of onset before 8 years of age. Source: U.S. Bureau of the Census. *The Blind and Deaf-Mutes in the United States: 1930.* Washington, DC: U.S. Government Printing Office; 1931.)

high of 67.5 per 100,000, in 1880, to a low of 32 per 100,000, in 1930.

Because of these wide variations—which the Bureau regarded as indicating flaws in its procedures—it requested that the U.S. Congress relieve it of the responsibility for collecting morbidity data in the decennial censuses required by the U.S. Constitution. Congress responded in 1956 by establishing the National Center for Health Statistics (NCHS) to determine "the health of the nation"—a task it continues to perform.[6]

Since 1971, NCHS's Health Interview Survey (HIS) has used the same methods to determine degree and age at onset of impaired hearing.[7] That methodological consistency makes comparisons between years straightforward.

Table 3.1 displays rates of hearing impairment gathered by NCHS's Health Interview Survey. Between 1971 and 1991, the prevalence rates for all hearing impairment (not deafness alone) increased from 6,900 to 8,600 per 100,000. When age-adjusted, the increase in the rate drops to 15%—still a substantial increase over a relatively short period of time.[8]

## Geographic Prevalence

The geographic distribution of hearing loss rates varies by nation, as well as within nations.[1] It is illustrated by two recent population surveys in adjacent countries: Canada, 1987, and the United States, 1991. The U.S. rate for hearing impairment was more than double that for its neighbor: 8,600 versus 4,100 per 100,000.[9] The 4-year difference in the time of each survey does not seem a likely explanation for so large a difference in the two rates.

Furthermore, using national data to estimate prevalence rates for divisions within each country yields similarly misleading results. The national Canadian average of 4,100 per 100,000 would be erroneous for most of its provinces, as shown in Table 3.2. Manitoba and Prince Edward Island had prevalence

**Table 3.1.** Rates of Impaired Hearing per 100,000 Persons 3 Years of Age and Older: United States, 1971, 1977, 1991

| Type of Prevalence Rate | Rates per 100,000 | | |
|---|---|---|---|
| | **1971** | **1977** | **1991** |
| Unadjusted | 6900 | 7000 | 8600 |
| Age-adjusted to 1991 | 7500 | 7300 | 8600 |

**Table 3.2.** Rate of Impaired Hearing per 100,000, by Political Division: Canada, 1987, and United States, 1991

| Subdivision | Rate per 100,000[b,c] |
|---|---|
| **CANADA**[a] | **4100** |
| Newfoundland | 4400 |
| Prince Edward Island | 6100 |
| Nova Scotia | 6000 |
| New Brunswick | 5600 |
| Quebec | 3400 |
| Ontario | 4700 |
| Manitoba | 6100 |
| Saskatchewan | 5000 |
| Alberta | 3800 |
| British Columbia | 4800 |
| Yukon | 3900 |
| Northwest Territories | 3400 |
| **UNITED STATES**[b] | **8600** |
| Northeast | 7100 |
| North Central | 9600 |
| South | 8800 |
| West | 8600 |

[a]Rates are for persons 15 years of age and older.
[b]Rates are for persons 3 years of age and older.
[c]Entries are rounded.

rates one-and-one-half times larger, whereas Quebec and the Northwest Territories had rates 20% smaller than the national average.

The continental United States reinforces the Canadian example of regional variability. The U.S. Bureau of the Census divides the country into four regions: Northeast, North Central,

South, and West. The 1991 prevalence rates for impaired hearing in these regions ranged from 7,100 per 100,000, in the Northeast, to 9600 per 100,000, in the North Central—more than a 35% difference (see Table 3.2).

The same prevalence hierarchy—highest in the North Central and lowest in the Northeast—has appeared in all prior decennial censuses of hearing loss in the United States, dating back to 1830.[10] Similar differences between regional prevalence rates have appeared in census data from other countries.[11]

## INCIDENCE

The ability to determine the number of new cases of hearing loss has improved in recent years. However, estimating incidence increases in difficulty as the age of a population segment increases—being easiest for newborns and most difficult for elderly persons.

The incidence of neonates with hearing loss at, and immediately following, birth has become increasingly available because of government actions (see "Infant Screening" in Section 1, Introduction). Although incidences will differ from place to place and over time, a typical rate for profound early deafness in school-age children has been found to range from 40 to 110 per 100,000.[12,13]

Contrary to prevalence rates, childhood and adult incidence rates of hearing loss are less available, in part, because they are not reportable conditions. Determining the number of new cases of late childhood and adult hearing losses arising in a specified time period is further complicated by fluctuations in individuals' hearing losses from near normal to severe, making it difficult to decide when or if to enumerate them, and by lack of agreement on definitions of hearing terms.

## POPULATION CHARACTERISTICS

Age, gender, and other demographic characteristics have shown correlations with hearing loss. The reasons for the relationships may appear simple though they are more likely complex, involving the compound effects of diseases, noise exposure, and injuries superimposed on individual genetics.

## Age

A plot of earlier prevalence rates for hearing loss in the United States appears J-shaped, a shape found repeatedly in various studies of age and hearing loss. Small proportions of the U.S. population had some degree of hearing loss up to about 50 years of age. After 50 years of age, the proportions increased sharply to a prevalence rate of about 15,000 per 100,000 for those 75 years of age and older (see Figure 1.3.1 in section 1.3).

More recently, a combination of studies based on audiologic examination and self-reports estimated that about a third of elderly persons 70 years of age and older had trouble hearing or were deaf in one or both ears. The study found "complete deafness" had prevalence rates for all ages combined from 5,900 per 100,000, in 1984, to 7500 per 100,000, in 1995.[14]

With the aging of the "baby-boom" generation, an increase in the proportion of the population with impaired hearing seems likely to rise rather than to decline or remain constant.[15] Since the average age of the U.S. population will likely continue to increase, it is reasonable to assume that the proportion of hearing loss in the population will also increase. Nonetheless, because aging alone does not account for the rate of hearing loss, other factors must be considered. One likely cause of increased hearing loss with age is noise exposure among young and middle-aged adults in the industrial populations.[16] Other factors likely to contribute to a greater prevalence of hearing loss are improved medical care for diseases and injuries that were previously fatal and expanded prescription of potentially ototoxic medications (see Section 1.2).

A caution: the relationship between age and hearing loss does not mean that aging *causes* hearing loss, a logically insupportable position as age refers to chronology not to a defined agent. Research to find the underlying mechanism—if one exists—has not so far succeeded, though ongoing investigations may yet find one or more genetic precursors.[17]

## Gender

Males are statistically at greater risk of impaired hearing than females. This generalization recurs in decennial censuses from 1830 to 1930, in recent surveys in the United States and Canada, in most studies of hearing impairment in other countries, and in virtually all studies of childhood deafness.[18,19]

With respect to degree of hearing loss, prevalence rates for severe and profound losses show males tend to exceed rates for females, as well as at lesser degrees of impairment. However, males appear to suffer greater losses in the higher frequencies and females in the lower frequencies.[20,21]

## Race, Ethnicity, Color, and National Origin

Race, ethnicity, color, and nationality have statistical relations to the prevalence of hearing loss. A persistent finding are higher rates of impaired hearing and deafness in Whites than non-Whites and lower rates in Whites than Hispanics and Asians. Prevalence per 100,000 for hearing loss has been found to be about 170 for African-American, 680 for Cuban-American, 280 for Mexican-American, 580 for Puerto Rican, and 160 for non-Hispanic white children.[22]

Canadian and U.S. findings are similar with respect to ethnicity. Whites in the U.S. have rates for impaired hearing that are about double those for non-Whites, whereas rates for Canadian Whites are almost five times greater than for non-Whites and nearly three times greater than for other minorities. Before accepting these findings at face value, it should be pointed out that the groups cited above differ in age-sex compositions, although these data are consistent with previous studies—all of which show Whites have higher rates of impaired hearing than non-Whites.[23]

Why these differences occur has been attributed to economic, genetic, and methodological explanations. None has been accepted as the single reason that explains the findings; indeed, it is likely the differences do not have a single explanation.[24]

## FAMILY COMPOSITION

Most deaf children come from nuclear families that have no deaf members. Multiple instances of deafness within a family tend to be the exception rather than the rule.[25]

### Parentage

The majority of deaf children in the United States have been raised by parents who have no personal experience with early-onset hearing loss. About 4% of deaf persons had deaf parents (3.2% with two deaf parents and 0.8% with one) in the United States, in 1971, compared with 3.3% of deaf persons with any deaf parents in the 1920 U.S. decennial census.[26]

The consequences of this mismatch between the hearing of parents and of their children have been probed. Deaf children born to deaf parents in the United States have been reported to have been better adjusted socially, tended to develop language more readily, and to do better educationally than their deaf peers from families with neither parent deaf.[27]

### Marriage

Preadult deafness has not been a bar to marriage, though the marriage rates among deaf persons tend to be lower than for the general population. In the three U.S. decennials, 1900 to 1920, rates of marriage for early-deafened adults compared to persons in general were found to be lower, although in each successive decennial the differential narrowed.[8] By 1971, a U.S. national survey found marriage rates for preadult deafened persons moving closer to the national average: 60% for deaf persons and 74% for the general population. Some of the lower marriage rates may be due to deaf persons tending to marry later than their age-peers in the general population; others may reflect inequalities in the composition of the comparison groups.[28]

Since early-deafened adults choose deaf marital partners at a ratio exceeding 9 deaf to 1 nondeaf, the lower marriage rates may also be due to limited choices of partners.[29] In the United States, at least 85% of individuals with profound deafness marry another deaf person—a high degree of assortive mating.

Gender differences also occur in marriage rates. Deaf males tend to have lower marriage rates than deaf females. As noted, because early deaf persons seek deaf partners, the fact that males constitute a larger portion of the deaf population than females presents a further limitation on marriages.[30]

## Birthrates

On average, the offspring of deaf-by-deaf matings have normal hearing. The rates vary somewhat by parents' ages at onset of deafness. Two prelingually deaf parents have been somewhat more apt to have deaf offspring than two later-deafened parents. But the majority of children born to deaf parents were not deaf.[31]

# ECONOMICS

Hearing impairment has not always attracted the U.S. government's financial support in proportion to its prevalence in the population. In 1970, U.S. deaf people were nearly four times more prevalent than those who were blind. Yet in that year, the U.S. Division of Vocational Rehabilitation (DVR) served 7,364 blind and 5,915 deaf clients. Had DVR's efforts been distributed in proportion to the relative sizes of the two groups, they would have served four times more clients who were deaf.[32]

## Employment

Hearing loss has not been an insurmountable bar to employment. Deaf adults tend to obtain jobs at rates close to those for the general population. However, comparable wage rates show a significant discrepancy that appears to reflect the fact that deaf persons tend to be passed over for promotions, particularly to supervisory and managerial positions, and persons who are hard of hearing often suffer similar discrimination.[33-35]

## HEARING AID USAGE

Among persons with sensorineural hearing loss, only about a fourth who might profit from amplification have it.[36] Despite revolutionary developments in portable and other forms of amplification, hearing rehabilitation reaches only about 1 out of 5 of Americans with significant auditory problems. Most of the remaining 4 out of 5 could profit from any of the presently available prostheses and audiologic procedures.[37]

## INSTITUTIONALIZATION

The preceding data relate to persons residing *outside* institutions. Rates for those who are institutionalized differ markedly from the general populations of which they are a part.

The U.S. National Nursing Home Survey, in 1985, found about 21% of institutional residents had impaired hearing.[38] A Canadian study in 1987 reported approximately 45% of Canadians residing in health-related institutions had impaired hearing. Clearly, persons in these institutions are more likely than the general population to have a hearing loss. But the two rates are not directly comparable: the United States limited its sample to nursing homes, whereas Canada included all health-related facilities. Differences in the way the two countries construe hearing impairment is also a likely factor in explaining the differences in the rates.

Audiometric surveys of prison populations also showed higher rates of impaired hearing in Canada than in the United States.[39] All together, then, persons who are institutionalized, regardless of the type of institution, have a higher probability of having a hearing loss than the general population of either country.

# TECHNICAL ISSUES

Although it may seem a simple matter, determining the sizes and characteristics of persons with hearing losses involves critical methodological decisions. The manner in which data are gathered can drastically skew results.

## Definitions

A great deal of the confusion about rates for hearing loss and deafness is due to conflicting definitions for the same terms. Deaf, according to some dictionaries, refers to "any loss of hearing" (Random House; Oxford). Hearing loss may be temporary or permanent; bilateral or unilateral; mild, moderate, severe, or profound. The reader facing contradictory rates must first determine if they all refer to the same entity.

Distinguishing between incidence and prevalence data is critical when digesting demographic information. *Incidence* refers to new cases arising in a unit time. *Prevalence* is the number of existing cases in a unit time. Adding together successive estimates of incidence, however, will not provide an accurate prevalence estimate. The reasons: some people were alive before the first incidence estimate, others die, some may be cured, and still others may leave the area. To determine either the incidence *or* prevalence of a condition at a particular place, in a given time period, requires studies to determine each statistic.

## Survey Versus Census

How the information about the number afflicted with a particular condition is gathered will affect the results. A census of a national population will likely produce results that differ from a special survey. The reason has to do with the mindsets of the persons being interviewed. Also, the design of a census usually does not allow for detailed inquiries needed to produce valid data.[40]

Procedures to determine the size of relatively rare populations embedded in large populations have been described.[41] The typical technique pairs register and survey to create a statistically powerful instrument. The availability of a tested register offers the additional advantage of yielding longitudinal and incidence data, something that the survey alone cannot provide.

## Assessing Hearing Ability by Interview

Two related but dissimilar methods of assessing hearing loss are (a) audiometry and (b) interviewing. The typical pure-tone audiometric examination asks the patient to indicate when a tone appears or disappears or to press a button. This interaction between an examiner and a patient resembles an interview, except that standard stimuli provide the basis for the patient's responses.

In an interview, patients are asked how well they hear, either in response to a single question or two or with respect to a verbal scale. The Hearing Ability Scale has been used by NCHS's HIS since 1968. Its relation to the audiometric pure-tone measure has been determined in the United States and Great Britain with virtually identical results: scale responses correlate highly with audiometric measures.[7,42]

## Combining Surveys and Registers

Registers of persons with a particular condition have been derided because of poor maintenance; for example, failure to expunge persons who no longer belong on it. Another difficulty is determining their completeness. To overcome the first objection only requires administrative diligence. The latter, however, incorporates a competing technique, the survey. A sample survey of the population identifies individuals who should be on the register, and multiplying their number by the sampling ratio yields an estimate of the number missing. This powerful procedure has further advantages, such as, being able to estimate incidence as well as prevalence.[39]

# SUMMARY

Studies of hearing impairment show that taking specific rates from one location or one time and applying them to another location or to another time will often lead to erroneous conclusions. The danger of such an exercise is shown by the comparisons between the recent U.S. and Canadian surveys of their citizens with impaired hearing. Prevalence rates not only vary between the two adjacent countries, but also from province to province and from region to region. Variations in rates occur from time to time, another finding amply supported by the data.

On the other hand, generalizations about hearing impairment and deafness frequently hold. Thus, almost every study finds that early deafness is a low-frequency condition, whereas overall hearing impairment regardless of age at onset is relatively frequent. How infrequent or infrequent depends on the location at a particular time. Because sample sizes on which some of these rates are based are small, we cannot say with certainty whether they reflect true changes or sampling variations. Other generalizations occur with such repetitiveness that even when based on small samples they appear valid. For example, it is safe to say that only a small portion of almost any sample will be prelingually deaf. Specifying how small a portion, however, is subject to substantial variation, geographically and chronologically.

The timeliness of data can be critical. Estimating the deaf and hard-of-hearing populations' sizes and characteristics is like trying to hit a moving target—one that not only changes speeds, but also zigs and zags. As illustrated by the NCHS data from 1971, 1977, and 1991 cited above, the relative sizes of the U.S. populations with impaired hearing have increased so rapidly that the rate from the earliest survey would miss the target by nearly 15%—a substantial change in only 20 years.

Broad statements about some demographic features appear well founded, changing only in their magnitude. Males are more likely than females to be hard of hearing and deaf. The older one becomes, the more likely one is to have impaired hearing. With respect to preadult deafness, the tendency of deaf people to take deaf spouses appears without exception in research reports. Likewise, the majority of deaf-by-deaf marriages have normal hearing, not deaf, offspring.

These generalizations have been found in many cohorts, locales, and time periods. They recur with regularity. Nonetheless, researchers should not stop studying them. They are not immutable; they could change, and their changes could be important. Methods that can track these changes by cost-effective means have been developed and tested. They await further applications.

# REFERENCES

1. Schein JD. 1973. Hearing disorders. In: Kurland LT, Kurtzke JF, Goldberg ID, eds. *Epidemiology of Neurologic and Sense Organ Disorders*. Cambridge, Mass: Harvard University Press; 1973:276–304.

2. Vision and Hearing Statistics. Access any year for current projections at http://www.cdc.gov/nchs

3. Schein JD, DeSantis V. Blindness statistics (Part I): an analysis of operational options. *J Vis Impair Blind.* 1986;80(1):517–522.

4. Schein JD, Delk MT. *The Deaf Population of the United States*. Washington, DC: National Association of the Deaf; 1978.

5. U.S. Bureau of the Census. *The Blind and Deaf-Mutes in the United States: 1930*. Washington, DC: U.S. Government Printing Office; 1931:1–32.

6. Vital and Health Statistics. Accessed for any given year at http://www/cdc/gov/nchs/data/series

7. Schein JD, Gentile A, Haase, K. Development and evaluation of an expanded hearing loss scale questionnaire. *Vital and Health Statistics.* 1970;2(37):1–24.

8. Ries PW. Prevalence and characteristics of persons with hearing trouble: United States, 1990–91. *Vital and Health Statistics.* 1994;10(188):1–46.

9. Schein JD. *Canadians with Impaired Hearing*. Ottawa, Canada; Statistics Canada; 1992:1–42.

10. Best H. *Deafness and the Deaf in the United States*. New York, NY: Macmillan; 1943.

11. Davis AC. The prevalence of hearing impairment and reported hearing disability among adults in Great Britain. *Int J Epidemiol.* 1989;18:911–917.

12. Marazita ML, Ploughman LM, Rawlings B, et al. Genetic epidemiological studies of early-onset deafness in the U.S. school-age population. *Am J Med Genet.* 1993;46:486–491.

13. Schildroth, AN, Karchmer, MA. *Deaf Children in America.* San Diego, Calif: College-Hill Press; 1986.

14. Desai M, Pratt LA, Lentzner H, et al. Trends in vision and hearing among older Americans. *Aging Trends No.2.* Hyattsville, Md: National Center for Health Statistics; 2001.

15. See projections issued by the U.S. Bureau of the Census for various periods at http://www.census.gov/projections

16. Miller MH. Hearing conservation in industry. *Curr Op Otolaryngol Head Neck Surg.* 1998;6(9):352–357.

17. Schein JD. Implications of hearing loss in the elderly population. *Hear Rehab Quart.* 1985;10(3):3–7.

18. Niskar AS, Kieszak SM, Holmes A, et al. Prevalence of hearing loss among children 6 to 19 years of age. *J Am Med Assoc.* 1998;279(14):1071–1075.

19. Schein JD. The demography of deafness. In: Higgins P, Nash J, eds. *Understanding Deafness Socially.* Springfield, Ill: Charles C Thomas; 1996:21–43.

20. Berger EH, Royster LH, Royster JD, et al. *The Noise Manual.* Fairfax, Va: American Industrial Hygiene Association; 2000.

21. Franks P, Bertakis KD. Physician gender, patient gender, and primary care. *J Womens Hlth.* 2003;12(1):73–80.

22. Wu C, Grant N. Asian, American, and deaf: a framework for professionals. *Am Ann Deaf.* 1997;142:85–89.

23. Access Silent Asia: America's First Deaf Asian Conference. September-October 1994. *Perspec Educ Deafness.* 1994; 13(1):1–5.

24. Stewart JL. Hearing disorders among indigenous peoples in North America and the Pacific Basin. In: Taylor OL, ed. *Nature of Communication Disorders in Culturally and Linguistically Diverse Populations.* San Diego, Calif: College-Hill Press; 1986:45–62.

25. Fraser GR. *The Causes of Profound Deafness in Childhood.* Baltimore, Md: Johns Hopkins University Press; 1976.

26. Schlesinger H, Meadow KP. *Sound and Sign: Childhood Deafness and Mental Health*. Berkeley, Calif: University of California Press; 1972.

27. Meadow KP. Socialization of deaf children and youth. In: Nash JE, Higgins PC, eds. *Understanding Deafness Socially.* 2nd ed. Springfield, Illinois: Charles C Thomas; 1996:71-95.

28. Schein JD. Effects of hearing loss in adults. In: Alberti PW, Ruben RJ, eds. *Otologic Medicine and Surgery*. New York, NY: Churchill Livingstone; 1988:885-910.

29. Rainer JD, Altshuler KZ, Kallman F, eds. *Family and Mental Health Problems in a Deaf Population*. New York, NY: New York State Psychiatric Institute; 1963.

30. U.S. Bureau of the Census. *Statistical Abstract of the United States.* Washington, DC: U.S. Government Printing Office; 1988.

31. Schein JD. *At Home Among Strangers*. Washington, DC: Gallaudet University Press; 1989.

32. Government allocations for vocational rehabilitation by disability. Retrieve for any year from http://www.nidcd.gov

33. Emerton RG, Foster S, Gravitz J. Deaf people in today's workplace: use of the ADA and mediation processes in resolving barriers to participation. In: Nash JE, Higgins PC, eds. *Understanding Deafness Socially.* 2nd ed. Springfield, Ill: Charles C Thomas; 1996.

34. Welsh WA, MacLeod-Gallinger J. Effects of college on employment and earnings. In: Foster S, Walters G, eds. *Deaf Students in Postsecondary Education*. New York, NY: Routledge; 1992: 37-61.

35. Bowe F, Schein JD, Delk MT. Barriers to the full employment of deaf persons in the federal government. *J Rehab Deaf.* 1973:6:1-15.

36. Miller MH, Schein JD. Improving consumer acceptance of hearing aids. *Hear J.* 1987;40(10):25-32.

37. Kirkwood D. Led by BTEs, sales rise for fourth straight year to surpass 2.3 million. *Hear J.* 2006;59(12):11,14-16,18, 20.

38. The Changing Profile of Nursing Home Residents: 1985-1997. Retrieved January 2000 from http://www.cdc.gov/nchs/aging act.htm

39. Jensema CK. Hearing loss in a jail population. *J Am Deaf Rehab Assoc.* 1990;24:49-58.

40. Schein JD. Does census make sense? *Disab Stud Quart.* 1990;10(3):17–18.
41. Hansen MH, Hurwitz WN, Madow WG. *Sample Survey Methods and Theory.* Vol I: *Methods and Applications.* New York, NY: Wiley; 1953.
42. Ward PR, Tucker AM, Tudor CA, et al. Self-assessment of hearing impaired adults in England. *Br J Audiol.* 1977;11:33–39.

# Author Index

## A

Aase JM, 136
Abadi RV, 58
Abbas PJ, 194
Abe S, 134
Abram HB, 179
Abrams H, 217
Afzelius BA, 58
Agnew J, 177
Ahmad, 135
Ahmed R, 62
Ål Dakhail AA, 140
Alberti PW, 61, 85
Ali A, 57
Allum JH, 198
Alpert JJ, 84
Altshuler KZ, 237
Ambrosetti V, 140
American College of Medical
    Genetics Expert Panel, 15
American Speech-Language-
    Hearing Association, x, 14,
    15, 132
Amsterdam JD, 158
Anderson G, 144
Anderson PJ, 56
Andreu AL, 60
Antenuis JC, 142

Anthony P, 145
Antonelli P, 199
Arbones, 135
Arlinger S, 178
Armour JAL, 63
Asif A, 57
Association of Late Deafened
    Adults, xi
Atkins JS, 177
Ator GA, 156
Attias J, 137
Atwood JL, 14
Auerbach-Heller L, 158
Avraham KB, 14
Ayache D, 144
Azevedo RB, 85
Aziz MH, 61

## B

Babu S, 86
Bachor E, 140
Baehring JM, 158
Bahmad F, 59
Bahram M, 138
Bai L, 16
Bailey S, 217
Baker KB, 132
Balaban Cd, 139

239

Baldwin MS.
Balk SS, 85
Balkany TJ, 86, 136, 199
Baloh RW, 157
Balsara NR, 215
Bamiou D, 132
Banister L, 88
Barakat AY, 63
Baratelli R, 199
Barker DF, 55, 60
Baron JA, 132
Barry KD, 177
Bartkiw B, 216
Bath Ap, 142
Bauer CA, 158
Baur B, 61
Bearer CF, 85
Beck AT, 143
Beck J, 144
Beck PH, 218
Beetzc R, 58
Bellis TJ, 141
Bellugi U, 218
Beltramello M, 135
Belyantseva IA, 85
Bentler RA, 178
Bequer N, 142
Berg AO, 15
Berger EH, 236
Bergman, 141
Berlin CI, 14
Berman S, 15, 86
Bernstein M, 217
Bertakis KD, 236
Best H, 235
Beyer DM, 216
Bijl RV, 217
Bilgin H, 136
Bilous RW, 63
Black FO, 157
Blake KD, 134
Blau A, 56
Bluestone CD, 87
Bodurtha J, 65

Boenki J, 157
Bojrab DI, 138
Bolabek W, 140
Boon H, 145
Booth J, 140
Bordelin J, 14
Botto LD, 61
Bowe F, 57, 237
Bowman GA, 217
Boyadjiev S, 55
Brackman DF, 195, 216
Brennan M, 218
Bretlau P, 139, 141
Brickley GJ.
Brockwell CW, 138
Brookhouser PE, 14, 86
Brooks DN, 88, 216
Brorsson B, 217
Brostoff LM, 87
Brown DL, 156
Brown G, 143
Brown JJ, 87
Brummett RE, 87, 145
Bruno C, 60
Buhler HC, 198
Bukauskas FF, 135
Bull PD, 142
Buller DB, 88
Burg JR, 87
Burgoon DN, 88
Bussoli TJ, 14
Byl FM, 137

**C**

Cahill LD, 196
Campbell KCM, 86
Cantekin EJ, 87
Carhart R, 140
Carmel S, 218
Carner M, 133
Carranza A, 142
Carter AS, 176
Carter NL, 86

Cartwright BE, 218
Cary R, 85
Cashin JL, 85
Casselbrant ML, 87
Castillo MP, 86, 142
Causse JR, 140
Chang EH, 134
Chang Q, 135
Charcot-Marie-Tooth
    Association, 55
Chasse T, 58
Chau C, 142
Chen C, 136
Chen DH-C, 16
Chen L, 86
Cheng AK, 199
Chernoff G.
Chess S, 84
Chevance LG, 140
Chin GY, 58
Chisholm TH, 179, 216
Chitayat D, 60
Choy D, 144
Christie PT, 57
Christodoulov P, 136
Chuong D, 14
Chute P, 198
Ciafaloni E, 59
Cienkowski KM, 176
Citron D, 216
Clark JG, 88, 176
Clark S, 85
Clarke-Lyttle J, 196
Cleaver VC, 217
Clemente B, 65
Coelho C, 145
Coffey R, 63
Cohen MM, 14, 65
Cohen NL, 194, 195, 199,
    200
Coker N, 196
Coletti V, 140
Colletti V, 133
Conlin AE, 137

Corchia C, 61
Cord MT, 178
Cornett RO, 218
Cortopassi GA 59, 87
Coulter D, 176
Cox TC, 56
Coyle B, 63
Crandall CC, 178, 215
Crane MA, 143
Cremers C, 56, 66
Cremers WRJ, 177
Cripps AW, 87
Cruickshanks KJ, 143
Crumling MA, 15
Cucci RA, 135
Cunningham C, 136
Curthoys IS, 158

## D

Dagan O, 14
D'Albora JB, 63
Dalton DS, 143
Dalzell L, 15
Damen GWJA, 198
Danner C, 138
Davenport S, 134
Davidson J, 61
Davies E, 145
Davis A, 143
Davis AC, 217, 236
Davis H, 16
Davis PB, 145
De Graaf R, 217
de Ruiter MM, 63
de Silva MG, 196
De Smet PAGM, 145
DeBella K, 60
Del Bo M, 140
Delacruz Å, 137
Delaney KA, 157
Delhorne LA, 179
Delie J, 85
Delk MT, 64, 235, 237

Dell'Osso LF,
deMiguel M, 135
Denise P, 134
Denjoy I , 58
Denoyelle F, 13
Derlacki EL, 140
Desai M, 236
DeSantis V, 237
Desmond AL, 158
Dettman SJ, 198
Devarajan P, 55
D'Hawse PD, 195
Dibonis DA, 179
Dieterich M, 158
Dietrich P, 141
DiGiovann JJ, 133
Dillon H, 177, 198
Dinces EA, 140
Dionisopoulos T, 13
Dionisopoulos T, 142
Dix M, 158
Djourno A, 194
Dobie RA, 143
Dodds, E, 137
Dodson H, 88
Donohue CL, 179
Dornhoffer JL, 138
Douek E, 88
Doweck I, 157
Dowell RC, 198
Down JHK, 135
Downs MP, 134, 136
Drachman DA, 159
Drew S, 145
Duggert P, 159
Dunn C, 197
Durant JD, 138
Durga J, 142
Dyson F, x

**E**

Earally F, 144
Eckstein JD, 53

Economides J, 136
Edwards BM, 134
Eiberg H, 56
Eichner JE, 55, 61
Eisenberg LS, 200
Elbax, 144
Elberling C, 216
Eldridge R, 60
Elliott MA, 142
El-Schahawi M, 58
Emerton RG, 237
Engelbert R, 63
English K, 217
Epley JM, 157, 194
Epstein CJ, 55
Epstein S, 16
Eriksen H, 59
Erler SF, 217
Escolar ML, 57
Esposito P, 62
Estabrooks W, 217
Etzel RA, 85
Eviatar A, 140
Eyries C, 194

**F**

Fabry D, 198
Facer JW, 138
Falk S, 88
Farfel Z, 56
Farmer J, 88
Fausti SA, 87, 88, 177
Fayad JN, 200
Fecther LD, 85
Feigenbaum A, 69
Fernandez PB, 84
Ferraro JA, 138
Fife TD, 157
Filip DJ, 55
Finnell JE, 145
Fiorino FG, 140
Fish JH, 61
Florina FG, 133

Forsline A, 176
Forstman BJ, 60
Foster S, 237
Fowler EP, 16, 84
Fowler KB, 84
Fox J, 143
Fozo MS, 61
Frankovich D, 58
Franks P, 236
Franz N, 142
Fraser GR, 14, 65, 236
French HT, 86
French JH, 84
Fria TJ, 142
Fried PA, 84
Friedman E, 56
Friedman JM, 60
Furman JM, 139


# G

Gabreels FJM, 59
Gacek MR, 157
Gacek RR, 157
Gagnier JJ, 145
Gannon JR, 219
Gantz BJ, 138, 146, 195, 196, 197, 199
Gapany-Gapanavicius B, 140
Garstecki DC, 217
Gatehouse S, 178, 216
Gates GA, 139
Geers AE, 179
Gelfand SA, 14, 55, 138, 141, 179
Gentile A, 235
Gersdorff M, 144
Gfeller KE, 195
Ghossaini SN, 136, 137, 139, 178
Giacino J, 89
Gifford RH, 195
Gilian C, 144
Gillinger M, 200
Girardi M, 158

Gist GI, 87
Glass JD,
Glassman SA, 15
Glorieux FH, 62, 63
Goeghegan PM, 88
Gold SL 144
Goldberg RB, 65
Goldstein B, 144
Golz A, 137
Gomaa NA, 197
Gomez-Hernendez JM, 135
Gordeon CR, 157
Gordon JS, 88
Gorga MP, 14
Gorlin RJ, 13, 65
Graham JM, 134
Grant N, 235
Grantham DW, 195
Gratto MA, 87
Gravel JS, 133
Gravitz J, 237
Gray L, 143
Gray WL, 144
Green GE, 135
Green JD, 139
Greisiger R, 198
Gresty MA, 138
Griffith A, 15
Grigorieva IV, 57
Gristwood RE, 140
Grolman W, 196
Gruen, PM, 142
Grundfast KM, 14
Guan M-X, 59
Gubbels SP, 197
Guererrio S.
Gupta A, 61


# H

Haase K, 235
Haddad RK, 84
Hain TC, 157, 158
Haines JL, 62

Hall JW, 56, 138
Halmagyi GM, 158
Halpin C, 136, 137
Hamel BCJ, 59
Hamiel OP, 55
Hamill TA, 139
Hanley PJ, 145
Hansen L, 56, 238
Hansen MR, 140
Harding B, 57
Harford E, 137
Harkins J, 218
Harno T, 136
Harris J, 61
Harrison M, 15
Hasegawa T, 63
Hasino E, 86
Haverkamp W, 58
Hawkins D, 217
Hazel JWP, 144
Hearing Loss Association of
    America, xi
Hecker EB.
Hefner MA, 134
Helt PV, 87
Helt WJ, 88
Henderson-Sabe J, 217
Henley CN, 87
Henry J, 89
Henry JA, 142, 143, 144, 145
Heppner C, 219
Herdman SJ,
Hertle RW.
Hertzberg V, 89
Herzfeld M, 216
Hesterlee S, 60
Hicks DE, 64
Hicks WM, 64
Hilal-Dandan R, 133
Hildebrand MS, 196
Himel HN, 133
Hinchliff R, 138
Hinger J, 198
Hirsch LM, 219

Hnath-Chisholm T, 217
Hoagland GA, 66
Hochenburger E, 85
Hodell Í, 145
Hoffman Brown ML, 84
Hoffman RA, 143
Hofmann S, 56
Holmes A, 236
Holstein-Rathlov N-H, 138
Hood JD, 138
Hood L, 133
Horlbeck D, 177
Horn CE, 133
Horoupian D, 64, 135
Horowitz A, 218
Hortnagel K, 56
Hosford-Dunn H, 14
Hotson JR, 157
House HP, 140
House WF, 132, 194
Howell SJ, 60
Hughes LF, 86
Huh M-J, 196
Hullar T, 176
Hunter CA, 57
Hurler G, 57
Hurwitz WN, 238
Hutchins TP, 59, 87
Huy PTB, 134
Huygen PLM, 57
Hyde ML, 61
Hynds PJ, 59

**I**

Ingraham CL, 65
Ioannidis JPA, xi
Ito Y, 63
Ízmanski M, 140
Izzo AD, 200

**J**

Jackler RK, 132, 216
Jacobson GP, 143, 158

Jacobson JT, 138
Jaffe B, 61
James K, 57
Jastreboff MM, 142
Jastreboff PJ, 144
Jenkins HA, 177
Jensema CK, 237
Jeong S-W, 196
Jerger J, 132, 141, 178, 200
Jervell A, 58
Jiang K, 55
Joachims HZ, 137
Johnsen NJ, 141
Johnson EE, 176
Johnson GI, 133
Johnson J, 89
Johnson JL, 14
Johnson R, 145
Johnsson LG, 141
Joint Committee on Infant
    Hearing, 15
Joki-Erkkila VP, 87

# K

Kagan A, 138
Kaiser-Kupfer MI, 60
Kaldo V, 144
Kallen HJ, 61
Kallman F, 237
Kalmar K, 89
Kalmon M, 16
Kamin BA, 87
Kammen-Jolly K, 61
Kamphoven JH, 63
Kantner G, 66
Kaplan LC, 56
Kapur YP, 84
Karas DE, 58
Karchmer MA, 84, 238
Karmody CS, 140, 142
Kartagener M, 58
Kasemsuwan S, 136
Kashgarian M, 58

Kasic J, 177
Katz FA, 84
Katz J, 14
Kearsey MJ, 55, 134
Keats BJB, 14
Keiser H, 136
Keith RW, 132
Kellerman A, 89
Kemink J, 196
Kerber KA, 156
Khan SY, 142
Khanim F, 56
Kieszak SM, 236
Kikuchi T, 134
Kileny PR, 134, 196
Killion MC, 176
Kim HH, 177
Kim L-S, 196
Kimber L, 65
Kimura RS, 134
King S, 200
King SM, 195
Kirchner C, 64
Kirk J, 56
Kirk KI, 200
Kirkham TH, 66
Kirkwood D, 237
Kisiel D, 179
Kisiel S, 179
Kitamura K.
Kjer, 56
Klerman GL, 89
Klipi T, 87
Koehler CM, 50
Kok D, 63
Konigsmark BW, 65
Konrad-Martin D, 88
Korf BR, 60
Korn SJ, 84
Kostovic I, 141
Kovach MJ, 65
Kramer LC, 219
Kreuger S, 217
Kricos PB, 142

Krmpotic-Nemanic D, 141
Kronenberg J, 199
Kuk F, 177
Kuller M 137
Kuszyk BS, 60
Kuypers W, 66
Kyd J, 87

# L

Lalwani AK, 16
Lamy M, 57
Land C, 63
Lange G, 139
Lange-Nielsen F, 58
Langereis MC, 198
Langman LW, 132
LaPorta R, 198
Latoo M, 60
Lawson DS, 200
League for the Hard of
    Hearing, xi
Lebo CP, 141
Lee H, 137
Lee KJ, 56
Lee SJ, 137
Lehmann MH, 58
Leigh J, 158
Leigh JR, 198
Leigh RJ, 158
Leigh-Paffenroth E, 88
Lempert T, 138
Lento CI, 200
Lentzner H, 236
LePage E, 86
Leprell CG, 86
Lesner SA, 142
Lesperance MM, 56
Leuenberger D, 59
Leung J, 199
Levitt H, 177
Lew H, 89
Liang S, 135

Liebermann F, 60
Lim HH, 133
Lin AE, 134
Lin D, 196
Lin J, 55
Linada-Grenada G, 13
Lindberg A, 60
Ling D, 216
Linstrom CJ, 61
Lipman RT, 144
Lipman SP, 144
Lipscomb DM, 86
Lisabeth LD, 156
Llanarz T, 133
Lm JG, 137
Loorin, 145
Lopez de Munain A, 58
Lowder MW, 197
Lucker JR, 216
Ludrigsen C, 177
Lummis RC, 194
Lustig LR, 64, 196
Luterman D, 195, 200, 215
Lutes-Driscill V, 218
Lutz R, 62
Luxford WM, 132
Luxon L, 132

# M

Maat A, 196
MacFarland W, 179
Maciel-guerra AT, 134
MacLeod-Gallinger J, 237
MacRae D, 13
Madow WG, 238
Mageroy K, 59
Mahan W, 178
Mainord JC, 139
Maki-Torkko EM, 217
Malinoff R, 179
Mann W, 139
Manthey D, 135

Marangos N, 198
Marazita ML, 236
Marcus DA, 139
Margolis RH, 217
Maroteaux P, 57
Maroudias N, 136
Marple BF, 140
Martin E, 139, 217
Martin FN, 88, 89, 176
Martin JL, 133
Martin JS, 141
Martin MM, 63
Mastroiacovo P, 61
Matkin ND, 15
Mattheis S, 177
Mattila PS, 87
Matz GJ, 85
Maurer, J 139
McArdle R, 216
McCabe B, 133
McCabe BF, 158
McDermott D, 57
McKenna MJ, 59
McKnight SL, 59
McMenomey SO, 197
Meadow KP, 237
Megalu UC, 145
Meijers-Heijboerb H, 58
Meilhle MB, 87
Melnick W, 85
Mendel LL, 217
Merchant SM, 59
Merchant SN, 59
Mestril R, 133
Metson R, 58
Meyer TA, 195
Meyerhoff WI, 136
Mhatre AN, 16
Mi Z, 63
Michael MG, 64
Michaels L, 86
Michel P, 132
Middleton A, 15

Migirov L, 199
Miller JM, 86
Miller MH, 16, 85 138, 143,
    178, 216, 236, 237
Mills R, 140
Mischke RE, 136
Mispagel KM, 177
Miyamoto RT, 200
Mohammed L, 60
Mohr J, 69
Molloy AM, 135
Montero M, 145
Moodie KS.
Moog JS, 179, 199
Morgan DW, 134
Morrrison Aw, 139
Mueller HG, 138
Mueller RJ, 55
Muller JM, 200
Munns C, 63
Murahashi K, 136
Muroya K, 63
Murty G, 63
Musiek E, 132
Musiek FE, 55
Myerhoff WH, 140

**N**

Nadol JB, 59
Nageris BJ, 137
Nair P, 133
Nance WE, 13, 55, 65, 134
Narcey P, 134
Nasher LM, 157
National Center on Low-
    Incidence Disabilities, xi
National Institute of
    Neurological Diseases and
    Stroke, 57
National Institute on Deafness
    and Other Communicative
    Disorders, xi

Naylor G, 216
Nazareth I, 156
Nemanic D, 141
Neubert WJ, 140
Nevins ME, 198
Newby HA, 141
Newman CW, 143, 145, 158
Newman NJ, 60
Newton VE, 65
Neyroud N, 58
Nguyen K, 60
Niedermeyer HP, 140
Niparko JK, 64, 196, 199
Nishimum HA, 143
Niskar AS, 236
Nixon CW, 85
Niyibizi C, 63
Noble W, 145
Noble W, 197
Noe CM, 216
Nolk E, 144
Nordahl D, 143
Northern JL, 89, 134, 216
Norton SJ, 14
Nouwen, J, 144
Novak KK, 132
Nussbaum D, 198

**O**

O'Leary VB, 135
Oh J-H, 137
Ohta R, 137
Oka Y, 59
Okamota M, 137
Oliveira CA, 144
Oliviera CA, 134
Olsson RT, 143
Online Mendelian Inheritance
    in Man, xi, 13, 56
Osaki Y, 143
Osberger MJ, 199, 218
Otto S, 195

Oviatt D, 196
Owen N, 156

**P**

Paki B, 145
Palmer CS, 199
Palmer CV, 217
Pan HWP, 140
Paparella MM, 136
Paradise HL, 87
Paradise JL, 142
Parfitt AM, 63
Parie-McDermott A, 135
Park K, 137
Parkinson AJ, 198
Parkinson DB, 63
Parnes, LS, 137
Parsa V, 177
Pasternak J, 133
Patel AM, 196
Pathria ESJ.
Patton MA,
Paul DI, 134
Paul M, 85
Paul PV,
Paul R, 142
Payad Jn, 137
Perez N, 139
Perry B, 60, 195, 196, 200
Perry BP, 146
Philliposian C, 134
Phillips DP, 132
Phillips DS, 88
Phillips JO, 157
Piazza V, 135
Piccirillo JF, 145
Pickett J, 179
Picton TW, 132, 133
Piel CF, 55
Piepmeier JM, 158
Pikus AT, 60
Pinckers A, 56

Pisoni DB, 198
Plauchie H, 13
Plotkin H, 62
Ploughman LM, 236
Poe M, 57
Poizner H, 218
Politzer A, 139
Post JC, 13
Prapsin BC, 196
Prasad S, 135
Pratt LA, 236
Preece JP.197
Presti PM, 61
Prieve B, 15
Primorac D, 62
Probst B, 59
Propst EJ, 196
Pruchno CJ, 35
Pryor SP.
Public Library of Medicine, x
Pulec JL, 139, 145

## Q

Quortrup K, 138

## R

Raas-Rothschild A, 55
Rabe, A, 84
Rabionet R, 135
Radke Å, 138
Rainer JD, 237
Rambold H, 157
Ranalli DN, 142
Raphael Y, 16
Rapin I, 13, 66, 87, 132, 133
Rauch F, 62, 63
Rauch Í, 137
Rauch SD, 136
Rawlings B, 236
Read AP, 65
Reavos KM, 88

Redell RC, 141
Reed CM.
Refaie A, 143
Regelein RI, 143
Reinhardt JP.
Reisinger KS, 84
Ret J, 196
Reuter G, 133
Riccardi VM, 61
Ricci E, 59
Ricketts TA, 177, 1944
Ries PW, 235
Rizer FM, 143
Ro A, 13
Roark R, 86
Robb NJA, 144
Robbins AM, 199
Robert E, 61
Robert KW, 134
Robinson B, 60
Rochon P, 145
Roesch K, 59
Roeser, RJ, 14, 15, 89
Rojeski T, 217
Roland JT, 199
Roland PS, 142
Roland PS, 86, 140, 199
Romo T, 61
Roscioli T, 56
Rosen S, 141
Rosenberg SI, 145
Rosenblum LD, 218
Ross M, 195
Rostgaard J, 138
Rouleau GA, 60
Roup CM, 178
Roush J, 15
Rowan PT, 145
Rowe D, 62
Royster JD, 236
Royster LH, 236
Royster, LH, 141
Ruben RJ, 58, 66

Rubenstein JT, 196, 197
Rubenstein LZ, 157
Rubinstein JT.
Ruckenstein MJ, 158
Ruffin CV, 198
Russell-Eggitt IM, 134
Rutter J, 59
Ryback L, 85, 87

# S

Sabo DL, 142
Sabo MP, 15
Sahud MA, 55
Sakkers R, 63
Saldana HM, 218
Salomon C, 141
Salvi PB, 87
Samy RN, 138
Sandlin RE, 143
Sando I, 136
Sandridge SA, 143, 145
Sano H, 137
Sarrazin AM, 58
Sartorato EL, 134
Sauerburger D, 218
Saunders GH, 176, 177, 179
Sauvaget E, 134
Saxena R, 55
Scalchunes V, 199
Schaap T, 140
Schachern PA, 136
Schechter MA, 143
Schein JD, 64, 85, 138, 141,
    194, 216, 218, 235, 236, 237,
    238
Scherl S, 62
Scheuerlla j, 142
Schiff N, 89
Schildroth AN, 236
Schlesinger H, 237
Schleuning AJ, 145, 146
Schneider ME, 85

Scholtz AW, 61
Schow RL, 215
Schuknecht HE, 141
Schultze-Bahr E, 58
Schum D, 216
Schwartz C, 59
Sclafani AP, 61
Scollie S, 142
Sedlimeier R, 140
Seewald RC, 142, 178
Segal J, 137
Seidman M, 86
Selesnick SH, 133
Selikowitz M, 135
Sengupta A, 142
Serra A, 158
Shallop JK, 195
Shannon RV, 195
Shanske S, 59
Shapport SM, 86
Shepard NT, 138, 157, 158
Shildroth AN, 84
Shinkawa H, 134
Shitara T, 137
Shoup AG, 15, 89
Shprintzen RJ, 65
Shulman A, 144
Sidey A, 176
Siebent JR, 134
Siegert R, 177
Sigaudy S, 142
Silverstein H, 145
Simmons FB, 194
Simmons, MA 86
Simon HJ, 177, 178
Sinclair ST, 178
Sininger Y, 132
Sinnathuray AR, 196
Sismanis A, 133
Sloper, 136
Smaldino J, 178
Smallbert, 143
Smedley TC, 215

Smith DW, 136
Smith RJ, 57, 134
Snik FM, 177
Sobiezczanka-Radoszewska L, 134
Sobrinho PG, 144
Sollman WP, 178
Sommer HC, 85
Soulier M, 142
Spitzer JB, 137, 178
Spitzer O, 157
Spivak LG, 15
Splawski I, 58
St John P, 14
Staab JP, 158
Staba SL, 57
Stach BA, 132, 141, 177
Stagno S, 84
Starr A, 132, 133
Stecker GC, 217
Stecker M, 198
Steed L, 145
Steel KP, 13, 14, 15
Steer RA, 143
Stein L, 133
Stewart DA, 218
Stewart JL, 236
Stockley TL, 196
Stool SE, 15
Stratigouleas ED, 195, 200
Straubhaar S, 198
Strauss KP, 218
Stritzke G, 157
Strom TM, 56
Strome SE, 132
Strong, BC, 135
Studen-Pavlovich DA, 142
Stuhl JS, 158
Su Y, 218
Sue CM, 60
Sugahara K, 86
Sullivan R, 219
Sullivan RF, 137

Surr RK, 178
Sweetow RW, 134, 217
Szudek J, 60

**T**

Takasawa M, 143
Takemoto T, 86
Tanakak K, 86
Tang W, 135
Tange RA, 61, 196
Tassabehji M, 65
Tearney L, 198
Teknos TN, 58
Telian SA, 158
Tesson F, 58
Thambisetty M, 60
Thelin JW, 134
Thomasis BD, 198
Thompson G, 15
Thompson T, 133
Thomsen J, 139
Thonnissen E, 135
Timothy K, 58
Toner JG, 196
Toricella H, 134
Toricello HV, 13, 65
Tos M, 139
Tranebjaerg L, 59
Travers R, 62
Tremblay K, 133
Trotter WR, 63
Tsukuda K, 59
Tucci DI, 139, 143
Tucker AM, 238
Tudor CA 238
Turman K, 62
Turner CW, 195, 199
Turner S, 136
Tuse RV, 139
Tye-Murray N, 215
Tyler RS, 143, 145, 194, 197, 216

# U

Ulanovski D, 137
United Mitochondrial Disease
  Foundation, 58
University of Iowa Health
  Care, 156
Upadhyaya M, 55
Urban BA, 60
Usami S, 134
U. S. Bureau of the Census,
  235, 237
Usher CH, 64

# V

Valente LM, 176
Valente M, 14, 137, 176, 177
Van Camp G, 134
Van den Hout JMP, 63
van den Oever-Goltstein MHL,
  198
Van der Wees J, 63
Van Hoesel RJM.
van Looij MAJ, 68
Van Looija MAJ, 58
VanRiper LA, 134
Varga R, 59
Vaughan N, 57
Venick V, 196
Venosa Ar, 144
Ventry I, 176
Verhodf P, 142
Vernon JA, 146
Vernon M, 65
Vidal C, 195
Vincent GM, 58

# W

Waardenburg PJ, 65
Wagener HP, 56
Walden BE, 178

Walford RI, 136
Waltzman SB, 199
Wang N-Y, 199
Wang S, 63
Ward PR, 238
Ward, WD, 141
Waslsh JT, 200
Watts JC, 55
Wazen JJ, 136, 137, 139, 178
Weber BA, 15
Wedekind H, 58
Weider DJ, 55
Weiner-vacher SR, 134
Weinstein B, 176
Weinstein BE, 141
Weiss AH, 157
Weissman MM, 89
Welsh LW, 64
Welsh WA, 237
Wetelecki W, 60
Wettke-Schafer R, 66
White KR, 14
Whitman GT, 137
Widen JE, 14
Wiet RJ, 140
Wijdeveld P, 56
Wilde RA, 145
Willecke K, 135
Williams HB, 13, 142
Willis HE, 133
Wilmington DJ, 87, 88
Wilson AC, 136
Wilson BS, 198, 200
Wilson PH, 144
Wilton P, 60
Winkel LP, 63
Wise CM, 133
Wiszniewski W, 134
Witt SA, 197, 198
Wladislavosky WP, 138
Wolf EG, 64
Wolfram DJ, 56
Woodall WG, 88

Wright D, 89
Wright E, 60
Wright JT, 140
Wu C, 236
Wyatt JR, 199
Wynne MK, 136

# X

Xu J, 84
Xu J, 84

# Y

Yakirevitch A, 16
Yalamanchili HR, 61
Yamasoba T, 59
Yanagita N, 137

Yardley L, 156
Yeagle JD, 199
Yellin MW, 139
Yerulkhimovich MV, 16
Yoo WN, 195
Yoshinaga-Itano C, 176
Yund EW, 178, 217

# Z

Zaghis A, 140
Zhang Y, 135
Zhou I, 138
Zimmerman-Phillips S, 196, 199
Zubieta JL, 139
Zuckerman BS, 84
Zuckerman BS, 84
Zwolan TA, 196, 198

# Subject Index

## A

Acid Maltase Deficiency
Association, 44
Acoustic desensitization
protocol, 129
Acoustic neuroma, 34
Acoustic trauma, 71, 82
  head injury, 82
  organic brain damage, 152
  prevention, 72
  stroke, 31, 81, 148
Adair-Deighton syndrome, 40
Aging of population. *See*
  Demography
Alabama Institute for Deaf &
  Blind, 214
Alaska Center for Blind and
  Deaf Adults, 214
Alexander aplasia. *See* Aplasia
  and Dysplasia
Alexander Graham Bell
  Association for the Deaf
  and Hard of Hearing, 214
Alpert syndrome, 20, 91
Alport syndrome, 9, 17, 91
Alprazolam, 130
Alstrom syndrome, 46

Amaurosis. *See* Blindness
American Academy of
  Audiology, 209
American Academy of Family
  Physicians, Joint policy
  statement, 76
American Association of the
  Deaf-Blind, 214
American College of Medical
  Genetics, 7
American Foundation for the
  Blind, 214
American Hearing
  Organization, 156
American National Standards
  Institute, 168
American Printing House for
  the Blind, 214
American Sign Language. *See*
  Sign languages
American Speech-Language-
  Hearing Association, 95,
  209
American Tinnitus Association,
  124
Americans with Disabilities
  Act, 174
Aminoglycosides, 18, 131

Amplification; *see also*
    Listening devices; Hearing
    aids
  anatomical/physiological
    considerations, 107
  conventional, 93
  sound-field, 175
Anophthalmia/Microphthalmia
    Registry 39
Anxiety disorders. *See* Tinnitus
Aplasia and dysplasia, 91
  Alexander, 91
  Michel, 91–92
  Mondini, 54, 91–92, 100,
    149
  Oto-spondylo-mega-
    epiphyseal dysplasia, 92
  Scheibe, 54, 92, 149
Aspirin. *See* Hearing loss
Assistive listening devices,
    174–175
  FM systems, 174
  hard-wired, 174, 211
  infrared, 175. 211
Association for Glycogen
    Storage Disease, 44
Association of Late Deafened
    Adults, 214
Atresia/Microtia Support
    Group, 39
Audiometry, 77–78, 233
  Bekesy, 81
  Conditioned Play
    Audiometry, 6
  conditioning techniques, 7
  delayed speech feedback, 77
  immitance testing, 71
  infant screening, 5
  interview, 233
  Lombard voice reflex, 81
  loudness recruitment, 77
  neurotologic history, 165
  otoacoustic emissions, 6, 71,
    81

  prefitting examination, 165
  stapedial reflex, 81
  Stenger, 81
  TROCA, 7, 79
  word-recognition, 77
  tympanometry, 77
Auditory brain implant. *See*
    Cochlear implant
Auditory brainstem response,
    81, 96, 171
Auditory dys-syncrony, 95
Auditory Integration Training,
    95
Auditory neuropathy, 95
Auditory Processing Disorder,
    118
Autoimmune disorders, 96
Autoimmune Inner Ear
    Disease, 96–98

# B

Bacterial infections. *See*
    Hearing loss
Balance disorders 152, 155; *see
    also* Dizziness; Vertigo
Behcet syndrome, 3
Bekesy audiometry. *See*
    Audiometry
Benign paroxysmal positional
    vertigo, 149, 154
Bibliotherapy, 215
Birthrates. *See* Demography
Blainville syndrome. *See*
    Oculo-Auriculo-Vertebral
    spectrum
Blindness, 46, 109
Bone-anchored cochlear
    stimulator. *See* Cochlear
    implant
Bone-Anchored Hearing Aid
    (BAHA). *See* Hearing aids
Branchio-Oto-Renal syndrome,
    91, 98–99

Brandt-Daroff exercises, 154
Brittle-bone syndrome, 39
Bruck syndrome, 40

# C

Canalithiasis, 149
Captioning, 210
Computer-Assisted Realtime
    Captioning, 210–213
Cued speech, 212
Cardiac arrhythmia. *See* Jervell
    and Lange-Nielsen
    syndrome
Cardiac disorders, 49
Cataracts, 9
Cayler syndrome, 49
Central Auditory Processing
    Disorder, 118
Cervico-Oculo-Acoustic
    syndrome, 52
Ceruman, 208
Charcot-Marie-Tooth
    Association, 19
Charcot-Marie-Tooth
    syndrome, 18
CHARGE Association, 2, 99
Children's Craniofacial
    Association, 39
Cholesteatoma, 75
Chromosomal anomalies. *See*
    Waardenburg syndrome
Cleft palate, 44, 49, 52, 122
Cochlear implant (CI), 96,
    181–194
  Advanced Bionics, 182
  age, 186–187, 189, 191
  anatomy and physiology, 185
  auditory brain implant, 184
  bilateral implantation, 187,
    194
  bioethics, 181
  bone-anchored stimulator,
    189

candidacy, 98, 184
  effects, side and long-term,
    187, 192
  future, 192, 194
  mechanical, 163
  Nucleus, 182
  Med-El, 182
  minimally invasive, 183, 193
  patient's health, 184, 186,
    192
  Penetrating Auditory Brain
    Implant, 184
  results, 180–191
  special populations, 162, 191
  tactile aids, 175
  team approach, 187, 190
  teenagers, 193
  variations, 183
Cognitive Rehabilitation
    Therapy (CRT), 129
Collagen, 39, 41
Communication supplements,
    210–213; *see also* Sign
    languages; Speechreading
  captioning, 210
  Computer-Assisted Realtime
    Captioning (CART),
    210–213
  Cued speech, 212
  fingerspelling, 212
  gestures, 211
  manual communication,
    211–212
  overhead projector, 211
  relay service, 210–211
  telecommunications, 210
Computerized dynamic
    posturography 151
Connective tissue disorder,
    122
Connexin 26 and 30, 10, 101
Contralateral Routing of
    Offside Signals (CROS).
    *See* Hearing aids

Counseling, 202–206
  educational, 202
  individual *versus* group, 206
Craniofacial dsyostosis, 20
Crouzon disease, 20
Cup ear, 36
Cupulolithasis, 149
Cytomegalovirus, 67

# D

Deafblind International, 214
Deafblindness, 46, 100, 210,
  213
Deafness. *See* Hearing loss
Demography
  age, 221, 227
  Baby-boom generation, 227
  birthrates, 230
  color, 228
  economics, 221, 230
  employment, 230
  ethnicity, 221, 228
  family composition, 229
  gender, 221, 232
  geography, 224
  incidence, 226, 232
  institutionalization, 231
  national origin, 228
  prevalence, 222, 232
  race, 228
  survey *versus* census, 232
  time, 232, 234
Desired Sensation Level
    formula. *See* Hearing aids
DFNA17, 185
Diabetes, 21, 208
  DIDMOAD, 21–22
DiGeorge syndrome, 24, 49
Disembarkment illness. *See*
    Dizziness
Disequilibrium. *See* Dizziness
Division of Vocational
    Rehabilitation, 214

Dizziness, 151, 154
  aging, 152
  Brandt-Daroff exercises, 154
  chronic, 152
  computer dynamic
      posturography, 151
  disembarkment illness, 149
  dysautonomia, 151
  ear rocks, 154–155
  Epley, 154
  imbalance, 149, 151–152
  mal de debarquement, 149
  otoconia, 154
  post-surgical, 149
  rehabilitation, 113
  stability testing, 151
  subjective, 152
  versus vertigo,151
Down syndrome, 102
Duane syndrome, 52
Dystonia-Deafness syndrome, 29

# E

Ear Popper, 75
Ear rocks. *See* Dizziness
EarCheck, 75
Ear wax, 208
Early intervention, 166
Edwards syndromes, 102
Eighth nerve (nVIII)
  auditory portion, 95
  neuropathy, 95, 150
  vestibular portion, 152
Ekman-Lobstein syndrome, 40
Electronystagmography. *See*
    Nystagmus
Electro-oculography. *See*
    Nystagmus
Electrotactile aids. *See* Hearing
    aids
Elephant Man's disease. *See*
    Neurofibromatosis
Employment. *See* Demography

Endolymphatic hydrops, 111
Epley maneuver. *See* Dizziness
Epstein syndrome, 18

## F

Fainting. See Jervell and Lange-
  Nielsen syndrome
FM systems, 174
Folic acid, 121
Food and Drug Administration,
  108
Fredreich ataxia, 30
Functional hearing loss, 80

## G

Gaining acceptance of
  amplification, 222–223
Gastric disorders, 152
GATA 3 mutations, 17
Gene manipulation as therapy,
  10
Genetics, 17, 91–92
  dominant, 92
  etiology, mixed, 92
  etiology, undetermined, 92
  molecular biology, 17
  recessive, 92
Geographic prevalence. *See*
  Demography
Gestuno. *See* Sign languages
Ginko biloba. *See* Hearing loss
Glue ear. *See* Otitis media
Glycogen storage disease, 43
Goiter, 42
Goldenhar syndrome, 35
Goldenhar Syndrome Support
  Network Society, 39

## H

Hard of hearing. *See* Hearing
  loss

Head injury. *See* Acoustic trauma
Health Interview survey. *See*
  National Center for Health
  Statistics
Hearing aids, 165–176
  Acclimatization, 173–174
  bone-anchored (BAHA), 107,
    172
  components, 167
  Desired Sensation Level
    formula, 172
  fitting children, 171
  fitting older patients, 172
  multichannel compression,
    169, 173
  prefitting examination, 215
  types
    analog *versus* digital, 168
    Bone-Anchored Hearing Aid
      (BAHA), 39, 107–108, 172
    behind-the-ear, 170–171,
      175
    body-worn, 170
    Contralateral Routing of
      Offside Signals (CROS),
      107–108, 172
    electrotactile, 175
    eyeglass, 170
    implantable, 169
    in-the-ear, 170, 203
    open canal, 203
    tactile, 93, 175
    ultrasonic, 162
    vibrotactile, 93, 175
Hearing conservation, 162,
  207–208
Hearing-ear dogs, 213–214
Hearing impairment. *See*
  Hearing loss
Hearing loss, 12
  Auditory Processing
    Disorder, 94, 118
  Autoimmune Inner-Ear
    Disease, 96–97

Hearing loss *(continued)*
  chemotherapy, 77
  conductive, 166
  congenital, 169
  degrees of, 12
  deafness, 12
  drugs and medications, 69,
    72
    alcohol, 69
    anti-nausea, 152
    aspirin, 78
    caffeine, 69, 151
    Ginko biloba, 130
    nicotine, 69
    recreational, 69
  incubator noise, 80
  infections, 67–68, 74, 208
    bacterial, 67
    Lues, 67, 81–82
    meningitis, 67, 69
    systemic, 152
    viral, 67, 148
  malingering, 80
    hysterical, 80
    nonorganic, 80
    pseudohypacusis, 80–81
    psychogenic, 80–81
    volitional, 81
  maternal behavior, 69
  maternal rubella, 68
  noise-induced, 69, 70–73,
    208, 227
  ototoxity, 76–79
  prematurity, 79–80
  sensorineural, 103
  sudden, 96, 104
  temporomandibular joint
    syndrome, 130
  trichloroethylene, 77
  unilateral, 9
  vascular insufficiency, 118,
    152
Hearing conservation, 208

Hearing Loss Association of
    America, 210, 214
hearing rehabilitation team,
    201–208
Helen Keller National Center
    for Deafblind Youth and
    Adults, 47
Hemifacial microsomia, 35
Hereditary Arthro-
    Ophthalmopathy, 122
Hereditary Motor and Sensory
    Neuropathy, 18
Heterochromia, 50
Hirschsprung disease, 51
Hunter syndrome, 23
Hurler syndrome, 23
Hypoparathyoidism-Deafness-
    Renal Dysplasia
    syndrome, 17, 24

**I**

Idiopathic sudden
    sensorineural hearing
    loss, 96, 104
Immitance testing. *See*
    Audiometry
Incidence. *See* Demography
Incidence in neonates. *See*
    Hearing loss
Incubator noise. *See* Hearing
    loss
Infant screening, 5, 171, 190
Infrared systems. *See* Assistive
    listening devices
Institutionalization. *See*
    Demography

**J**

Jensen syndrome, 30
Jervell and Lange-Nielsen
    syndrome, 25–26

Joint Committee on Infant Hearing, 5–6
Kabuki syndrome, 91, 93
Kartagener syndrome, 26
Kearns-Sayre syndrome, 28
Keratitis-Ichthyosis-Deafness syndrome, 109
Kidney disease, 17, 24

## L

Labyrinthitis. *See* Vestibular disorder
Lactic acidosis, 31
Lip reading. *See* Communication supplements
Listening and Communication Enhancement Program, 207
Lombard voice reflex. *See* Audiometry
Lop ear, 36
Loudness recruitment. *See* Audiometry
Lysosomal-storage disorder. *See* Pompe disease
Lues, 81–82

## M

Mal de debarquement. *See* Dizziness
Malingering. *See* Hearing loss
Mandibulo-Facial Dysostosis, 44
Manual communication, 211–212; *see also* Sign languages
  fingerspelling, 212
  gestures, 211
March of Dimes, 104
Marriage. *See* Demography
Marshall-Stickler syndrome, 122

Masking. *See* Audiometry
Maternal behavior during pregnancy. *See* Hearing loss
Maternal rubella, 67–68
Medication. *See* Hearing loss
MELAS syndrome, 30
Melatonin supplementation. *See* Tinnitus
Meniere disease, 81, 96–97, 110; *see also* Vertigo
  Meniett device, 114
  migraine, 112
Meningitis. *See* Hearing loss
Michel aplasia. *See* Aplasia
Migraine. *See* Meniere disease
Mitochondrial disease, 28
  Kearns-Sayre syndrome, 28
  Mohr-Tranebjaerg syndrome, 29
Mohr-Tranebjaerg syndrome, 29
Mondini dysplasia, 54, 100
Muscular Dystrophy Association, 44
MYH9 mutation, 185
Myozyme (alglucodidase alfa). *See* Pompe disease
Myringotomy, 75

## N

National Ambulatory Medical Care survey, 148
National Association of the Deaf, 214
National Captioning Institute, 210
National Center for Health Statistics, 148, 221, 223
National Center for the Study and Treatment of Usher syndrome, 47

National Hearing Conservation
  Association, 214
National Institute of Deafness
  and Other Communicative
  Disorders, 94, 98, 150
National Institute of Health, 33
Nausea. *See* Vertigo
Neonatal screening. *See*
  Audiometry
Neurofibromatosis, 32
  Elephant-Man's disease, 32
  Type II, 32, 186
Neuromonics tinnitus
  treatment, 129
Newborn auditory screening.
  *See* Audiometry
Nicotine. *See* Hearing loss
Nilkawa-Kuroki syndrome, 91
Noise-induced hearing loss.
  *See* Hearing loss
Norrie disease. 34–35
Nystagmus, 150, 153, 155
  electro-oculography, 151
  print reading, 155–156

# O

Ocular disorders. *See*
  Blindness; Nystagmus
Oculoauicular dysplasia, 35
Oculo-Auriculo-Vertebral
  spectrum, 35
Online Mendelian Inheritance
  in Man, ix
Onset of deafness. *See* Hearing
  loss
Optic atrophy. *See* Blindness
Organic brain damage. *See*
  Acoustic trauma
Organizations; *see also*
  individual organizations
  self-help, 214
  government, 214

  voluntary, 214
Ossicular chain, 20, 75, 169
Osteogenesis imperfecta, 39
Otitis media, 73–76
  adhesive, 75
  glue ear, 75
  Kartagener syndrome, 26
  middle-ear effusion, 73, 76
  serous, 73
  ventilation tubes, 75–76
Otoacoustic emissions. *See*
  Audiometry
Otoconia. *See* Dizziness
Otolaryngology Clinical Trial
  Cooperative Group, 96
Otologic's MET Fully-
  Implantable Ossicular
  Stimulator, 169
Otosclerosis, 114, 121
  clinical, 116
  histological, 115
  sodium fluoride, 117
Oto-spondylo-megaepiphyseal
  dysplasia, 122
Otospongiosis, 114
Ototoxic medications. *See*
  Hearing loss

# P

Patau syndrome, 102
Pendred syndrome, 42, 54, 92
Pep-net, 174
Peroneal Muscular Atrophy,
  18
Phytanic-acid-storage disease,
  46
Pierre Robin sequence, 122
Point-light technique. *See*
  Speech reading
Pompe disease (PD), 43
Positional/postural dizziness.
  *See* Dizziness

Postural instability. *See* Dizziness
Prefitting examination. *See* Audiometry
Premature birth. See Hearing loss
Presbycusis, 2, 31, 117
Prevalence. *See* Demography
Primary ciliary dyskinesia, 58
Pseudohypacusis, 80, 81
Psychogenic hearing loss. *See* Hearing loss
Public Health Service Guidelines, 8

**Q**

QT-arrhythmia syncope. *See* Jervell-Nielsen syndrome

**R**

Refsum syndrome, 46
Reissner's membrane, 93
Renal dysfunctions, 17–18, 98

**S**

Scheibe aplasia. *See* Aplasia and dysplasia
Sedlaakova syndrome, 49
Self Help for Hard of Hearing People, 214
Semicircular canal malformations, 47
Serous otitis media, 73–74
Shahl's cup. *See* Oculo-Auriculo-Vertebral spectrum
Shprintzen syndrome, 49
Sign languages, 211–212
   American Sign Language, 212
   Gestuno, 212

Spectrum, 35
Speech conservation, 207–208
Speech reading, 162, 209
   Point-light-technique, 209
Stability testing. *See* Dizziness
Stapedial-reflex. *See* Audiometry
Stenger test. *See* Audiometry
Stickler syndrome, 122
Syndrome, 1
Syndrome vs. sequence, 12
Syphilis. *See* Lues
Systemic infections. *See* Hearing loss

**T**

Tactile aids. *See* Cochlear implants; Hearing aids
Tangible Reinforcement Operant Conditioning Audiometry, 7
Telecommunications. *See* Communication supplements
Tinnitus, 2, 76, 78, 83, 115, 124–130
   anxiety, 125
   biofeedback, 130
   cognitive rehabilitation therapy, 127
   inventories, 126–127
   masking, 128
   melatonin, 130
   Neuromonics retraining therapy, 120, 129
   objective, 125
   pulsatile, 125
   residual inhibition, 129
   subjective, 124–125
   temporomandibular joint syndrome, 130
Xanax, 130

Traumatic brain injury, 82
Treacher-Collins Foundation, 45
Treacher-Collins syndrome,
    44–45, 92
Trisomy aberrations, 102
Tympanometry. *See*
    Audiometry

# U

U. S. Bureau of the Census,
    222, 225
U.S. National Nursing Home
    Survey, 231
Usher syndrome, 9, 46–47, 100
Van der Hoeve syndrome, 40
Velocardiofacial syndrome, 49
Ventilation tubes. *See* Otitis
    media
Vertigo, 96, 155; *see also*
    Tinnitus
  dysautonomia, 153
  essential, 152
  nausea, 152
  subjective, 152

# V

Vestibular Aqueduct
    Malformations (VASCM),
    47; *see also* Semicircular
    canal malformations
Vestibular disorders, 149; *see
    also* Dizziness; Eighth
    nerve; Vertigo
  chronic, 100, 149
  defined, 147

disequilibrium of aging, 149
  labyrinthitis, 130, 150
  post-surgical imbalance, 149
  rehabilitation, 154–155
Vestibular Ear Disorder
    Association, 156
Vestibular neuritis. *See* Eighth
    nerve
Vestibular system, 147
Vestibulopathy. *See* Vestibular
    disorders
Vibrotactile aids. *See* Hearing
    aids
Viral infections. *See* Hearing
    loss
Von Recklinghausen's disease,
    32, 162

# W

Waardenburg syndrome, 50,
    54, 92
Waardenburg-Shah syndrome,
    51
Ward-Romano syndrome, 26
Web feet, 20
Wildervanck syndrome, 52, 92
Wolfram syndrome, 21
World Federation of the Deaf,
    212
Worldwide Society of Wolfram
    Syndrome Families, 22

# X

Xanax. *See* Tinnitus
X-linked inheritance, 53